WOMEN UNDER THE KNIFE
A Gynecologist's Report on
Hazardous Medicine

To my father, Morris Keyser, the most honest, ethical, loving individual I have ever known, and to the many dedicated and brilliant physicians who have trained and inspired me to attempt to reach the high standards they have set.

women under the knife

A Gynecologist's Report on
Hazardous Medicine

Herbert H. Keyser, M.D.

Associate Clinical Professor of Obstetrics and Gynecology
University of Texas Health Sciences Center
San Antonio, Texas

A People's Health Library Book
Edited by Stephen Barrett, M.D.

George F. Stickley Company
210 West Washington Square
Philadelphia, PA 19106

The People's Health Library is a series of easy-to-read books written by experts who explain health and health care concepts for the general public. For a complete list of titles, send a self-addressed, stamped envelope to the George F. Stickley Company, 210 West Washington Square, Philadelphia, PA 19106.

Manufactured in the United States of America; Published by the George F. Stickley Company, 210 W. Washington Square, Philadelphia, PA 19106.

CONTENTS

ACKNOWLEDGMENTS

This book could never have been completed without the help of many people.

I want to thank my editor Dr. Stephen Barrett, who challenged me for over a year to think and re-think every statement and conclusion, George and Margot Stickley who had the faith and confidence to believe in the ideas I wanted to present, a large number of brilliant and highly ethical physicians who took the time to review, criticize, and recommend changes in the manuscript, to Bonnie Cummings and Cheryl Niles who worked diligently for hours to type and re-type; finally to my dear and precious wife Barbara for her understanding, support, and love which was so necessary in view of the personal and professional stresses which have been created by the decision to come forth with this information.

PREFACE

This book describes certain irresponsible practices which I have observed during more than 20 years in my specialty of obstetrics and gynecology. During my first 12 years of training and private practice, I took it for granted that medicine—like virtually every other profession—had a few bad apples. Then I became co-director of a department of obstetrics and gynecology at a large hospital in New York. Having access to data concerning large numbers of patients, I saw for the first time how significant a small number of bad apples can be—when they do surgery. Thus began my research, which has continued for more than a decade.

Although this book reveals some frightening facts about the "business" of medicine, I must stress that it is not intended to be a sensational expose. I certainly do not believe that most physicians are charlatans or that consumers can protect themselves from the "evils" of present-day medicine only by extraordinary or deceptive means. I wish merely to detail some of the problems of medical practice today: the economic, emotional and political factors which underlie certain abuses, and the difficulties inherent in weeding out hazardous practitioners. I will also try to outline the rational means (including the use of second opinions) by which women can obtain responsible medical care, for there is no question that the best defense against hazardous medicine is *knowledge*.

Abuses within the profession have led the government to mandate professional review boards to monitor the activities of physicians receiving funds through Medicare and other federal agencies. Most hospitals have set up internal committees to oversee length of hospital stay, utilization of resources, investment in costly equipment and other standards by which the profession may be judged. While these efforts should eventually result in overall improvement within the profession, even stronger measures will be needed to weed out the very small group of unethical physicians who knowingly or unknowingly deceive the public.

Women who read this book should find it helpful in evaluating their obstetrical and gynecological care. I hope that doctors who read it will search their conscience to determine whether the many stresses of modern medicine have ever led them to engage in hazardous practices. Equally important, have they observed questionable medical practices by others—and remained silent instead of speaking up?

Herbert H. Keyser, M.D.

Methodist Plaza
4499 Medical Drive
San Antonio, TX 78229

ABOUT THE AUTHOR

Herbert H. Keyser, M.D., is certified by the American Board of Obstetrics and Gynecology and has practiced his specialty for more than 20 years. He is a fellow of the American College of Obstetricians and Gynecologists and the American College of Surgeons. A 1958 graduate of Hahnemann Medical College in Philadelphia, he completed his internship and specialty training at Brookdale Hospital, Brooklyn, New York, and entered private practice in Merrick, Long Island, in 1963. For more than ten years he was deeply involved in developing Family Life Education programs and in women's and civil rights activism. In the late '60s, he served as a Lt. Colonel in the U.S. Army, after which he became active in the anti-Vietnam War movement.

From 1970 through 1978, Dr. Keyser was Director of Obstetrics and Gynecology at a large community hospital on Long Island and Assistant Professor of Clinical Obstetrics at State University of New York at Stonybrook. Since 1978 he has been Associate Clinical Professor of Obstetrics and Gynecology at the University of Texas Health Sciences Center, San Antonio, where he is also in private practice. His special interests include infertility and human sexuality. He has written numerous articles in medical journals and books. He and his wife, Barbara, reside in San Antonio and have six grown children.

ABOUT THE EDITOR

Stephen Barrett, M.D., a practicing psychiatrist and nationally renowned consumer advocate, is author/editor of 16 books, including *The Health Robbers* (a comprehensive expose of quackery), *Vitamins and "Health" Foods— The Great American Hustle, Shopping for Health Care,* and the college textbook *Consumer Health—A Guide to Intelligent Decisions.* An expert in medical communications, he is medical consultant to WFMZ-TV, Allentown, Pa., Editor of *Nutrition Forum* newsletter, and Consumer Health Editor of *Nautilus Magazine.* He is also a scientific advisor to the American Council on Science and Health and serves as Consulting Editor of its bimonthly newsletter.

FOREWORD

Women Under the Knife is not an "anti-doctor" book. Quite the contrary. Without sensationalism, Dr. Keyser presents to both patients and doctors a sober, thoughtful and informative work—free of medical jargon—intended to help those who wish to preserve a warm, mutually respectful, productive and confidential patient-doctor relationship.

The discussion is limited to Dr. Keyser's areas of expertise, obstetrics and gynecology. He is careful to emphasize that his criticisms are aimed at a relatively small number of fellow practitioners. Observations from his extensive clinical experience and personal research are fortified by statistics and published statements from well known and respected leaders representing the highest echelon of the medical establishment.

Women will find within this book sophisticated advice on avoiding unnecessary procedures and selecting trustworthy physicians. Doctors, it is hoped, will be inspired

Dr. Spain, a prominent forensic pathologist, was Professor of Clinical Pathology at Columbia College of Physicians and Surgeons, Chief Medical Examiner of Westchester County, New York, and a member of the New York State Board of Medicine and the State Professional Conduct Committee.

to look more closely at some of their own habits of practice as well as those of their errant colleagues.

From years past I recall a quote in the preface to a text on the history of medicine: "Only a good person can become a good doctor." Dr. Keyser is such a person and serves as a good doctor in a specialty whose past is replete with bad things done to women by bad doctors.

David M. Spain, M.D.

FOREWORD

Herbert Keyser deserves our gratitude for his courage and dedication. He has written an outrageously frank book that holds a mirror up to physicians, particularly obstetricians and gynecologists. He rightly points out that far too many D&Cs, cesarean sections, hysterectomies and breast operations are being performed. Like Job, who spoke of "physicians of no value," he emphasizes that the small proportion who are to blame put a stigma of distrust on the rest of us.

This book will no doubt irk many in the medical profession, especially those who suffer from that insidious disease, *furor operativa*, but Dr. Keyser asks us to take stock and improve regulation of our practices before the government steps in and tries to do it for us.

Books like this are needed to sensitize physicians to a higher conscience. It is not too late.

Robert B. Greenblatt, M.D.
Professor Emeritus of Endocrinology
Medical College of Georgia

1

HAZARDOUS
MEDICINE

The thesis of this book is simply stated: a small but significant number of gynecologists are driven by ignorance, impatience, indifference or greed, to practice hazardous medicine.

What do I mean by "hazardous medicine"? For patients it translates into unnecessary surgery, or to simple office procedures being needlessly transformed into costly hospital-based operations. For the public, it contributes to soaring health care costs and a pervasive sense of uneasiness about the ethics of the medical profession. These issues—which are quite complex—present an awesome challenge to both physicians and consumers.

I specialize in the practice of obstetrics and gynecology in San Antonio, a bustling city of almost one million people, where the vast majority of physicians are well-trained, responsible and competent. There are, however, some who are driven by ego or other private demons to practice hazardous medicine.

A "friendly" call

Not long ago, my secretary announced a telephone call from a local physician whom I'd met several times at social and medical functions. As far as I knew, he enjoyed a good professional reputation and was well liked by his patients. After we chatted for a while about subjects of mutual interest, he got down to the purpose of his call.

He wanted to talk to me "as a friend," he explained, because a patient of his was scheduled to see me the following week. She was being referred by her insurance company for a second opinion concerning his recommendation that she undergo a hysterectomy. "We doctors have to stick together," he said. "It's the only way we can beat the insurance companies at their own game."

At that point the purpose of his call was clear. He wanted me to concur with his decision to remove the uterus of Mrs. A, a 33-year-old patient whom he had been treating for several years for recurrent infection of the vagina. At one time a Pap smear had been slightly abnormal because of cervical inflammation, but subsequent Pap smears had been normal. Mrs. A, who wanted no more children, had been using birth control pills for more than four years. (These pills can sometimes make women more prone to certain vaginal infections.)

Why did he think she needed the operation? My colleague's explanation seemed a bit muddled. Her only real problem was the recurrent infection. Although that type of problem can be uncomfortable, it is not dangerous. It is certainly no reason to have a hysterectomy.

Of course, my colleague did not frame the patient's complaint so baldly. He led me through vague suggestions of other possible reasons for surgery, such as contraceptive failure and excessive bleeding. He concluded his telephone call by reminding me of an upcoming meeting of our obstetrical society, a none-too-gentle hint that we shared a common professional bond.

I was wary, but decided to withhold comment until I'd examined the patient and her medical records. Mrs. A's physical examination was normal except for an inflammation of the cervix with a moderate amount of creamy white discharge due to bacterial infection. The records from the gynecologist, which were quite detailed, contained no mention of excessive bleeding.

After my review was completed, I felt appalled. My colleague was attempting to pressure his patient into a major operation although he knew better. Mrs. A, an intelligent woman quite capable of weighing the pros and cons of treatment alternatives, had not been given the facts needed to make an informed choice. Rather, she had been advised that a hysterectomy was the appropriate way to eliminate the infections, and, as an added benefit, to end her fertility. As a result of this advice, she was prepared to undergo *major surgery* with little understanding of the risks involved.

The doctor had suggested that a hysterectomy was the *only* way her infection could be controlled. This was simply untrue. Moreover, he should have done several things which had been neglected. The cervix is at the tip of the uterus which projects into the top of the vagina. Its position in a dark, warm environment, as well as the normal trauma it sustains during the process of childbirth, makes it a natural site for chronic inflammation. Other factors— the bacteria that normally live in the vagina, vaginal acidity and birth control hormones—can all be involved in a causative way.

Mrs. A's gynecologist could have cleared up the cervical inflammation with local cryotherapy (freezing) or cauterization (burning), simple office procedures that take no more than a few minutes. Since vaginal infections may pass back and forth between sexual partners, the doctor should have obtained vaginal cultures or examined a smear under the microscope and treated the patient and her husband with appropriate medication. Finally, he might have stopped the birth control pills and advised use of mechanical devices such as condoms with foam or a diaphragm with contraceptive jelly. Or, if the patient wished to do something permanent to avoid pregnancy, she or her husband could be sterilized with methods much safer and less expensive than hysterectomy.

Of course, I advised Mrs. A not to have a hysterectomy and outlined my reasons for suggesting a more conservative approach. I presented these ideas very carefully to avoid undermining her longstanding relationship with the gynecologist. My letter to the doctor was completely professional in outlining the reasons for my nonconcurring second opinion. I included all of my recommendations without speculating about how or why he had reached his conclusions.

When I returned to my home that evening, did I experience the sense of a job well-done—a feeling that I had contributed to the welfare of my fellow humans? I did not, and the reasons for my dissatisfaction are in many ways my reasons for writing this book.

Misplaced trust

I sensed that Mrs. A would not follow my advice. She had complete trust in the doctor who had taken care of her for many years. She wanted a definitive solution to her complaints; and I had recommended against the surgery that to her appeared to offer such a solution. In the light of her trust, my concern about the hazards, expense and inappropriateness of major surgery seemed only to confuse her!

To make matters more complicated, if she proceeded with surgery, Mrs. A would in all probability wind up delighted with the results. She would have no further problem with contraception, even though there was no question that her fertility could easily have been controlled by other far less drastic means. Though hysterectomy is never a treatment for vaginitis, those symptoms would probably have disappeared in exactly the same way that local vaginal medication and some change in her contraceptive practices would accomplish. Excessive bleeding, which in young women can be due to everything from stress to temperature changes, would also have been controlled.

But it must be emphasized that no surgical procedure is without risk of death, surgical injury, hospital-based infection, or other serious mishap. Death or disability from unnecessary surgery is not merely tragic—it is unconscionable! Mrs. A did not need major surgery. Had she been informed by her own doctor of the risks involved, she might have decided against it. In fact, were it standard policy to obtain a second opinion, patients might be better able to approach second opinions with an open mind.

This incident illustrates some of the intricacies of hazardous medical practice which are discussed in this book. It also illustrates why I believe that elective (non-emergency) surgery should *rarely* be undertaken without a competent second opinion. I wish I could say that Mrs. A's case is an isolated or extreme example of hazardous medicine. Unfortunately, I have seen many during my years of medical practice.

Why women are vulnerable

At least ten factors contribute to the problem of hazardous medicine:

1. *Patients are anxious and uncomfortable.* It is human nature to seek relief from one's discomfort. It is also human nature to expect that doctors, most of whom are well-trained and ethical, will give trustworthy advice. But overanxious patients sometimes push doctors into operating against their better judgment.

2. *Many decisions fall into "gray areas" where the best course of action is not clear-cut.* In such cases, weighing the benefits of surgery against the possible risks can be very complicated. For example, sometimes a medical alternative to surgery is safer and less costly, but takes longer or is less certain. For example, as noted in Chapter 5, the fear of being sued for malpractice is driving doctors to perform cesarean sections that are medically unnecessary.

3. *Doctors are anxious to help their patients become comfortable as quickly as possible.* While this is a desirable attitude, it can sometimes induce doctors to suggest radical action which offers quick relief rather than conservative action which is safer but takes longer.

4. *Some procedures are far more lucrative than others.* Thus in close decisions—or even in some which are not close at all—financial factors may influence the doctor's choice of method.

5. *Consumers cannot always be well-informed.* The less sophisticated the patient, the more vulnerable she is. A patient may lack the time, interest, background or training needed to research medicine or even her own problem

adequately. Should we fault those who rely primarily on their doctor's reputation?

6. *Even well-informed patients can have difficulty in detecting poor medical judgment.* Patients are unlikely to become so sophisticated that they can out-think the average doctor. Moreover, some surgical decisions must be based upon observations available only to the doctor—such as the appearance of the patient's cervix, the size and shape of the uterus, or whether an expectant baby is showing dangerous signs of distress.

7. *Many doctors who recommend unnecessary surgery have very good reputations!* It is a sad but essentially valid maxim that surgeons are almost never chastised for doing unnecessary procedures; they get into difficulty only if they do their work poorly. The unfortunate corollary to this is that the physician who does a great deal of unnecessary surgery is usually technically very skillful. If he were not, a mounting number of malpractice suits would soon force him into a more conservative stance. This is why patient protection ultimately lies within the medical profession. Some unethical behavior can be detected only by professionals who have equivalent training.

8. *What takes place in a doctor's office is private and rarely subject to peer review.* Second opinion programs can overcome some of this difficulty, but most doctors don't favor them. Most doctors who write on this subject conclude that second opinions should not be required, and that unnecessary surgery is rare. I disagree.

9. *In many hospitals, peer review is not working well.* Although peer review mechanisms exist whereby doctors review each others' work, in many areas they are not functioning effectively. All accredited hospitals have committees responsible for judging the appropriateness of surgery in their institutions. But not all committee members approach their tasks with zeal.

In voluntary nonprofit hospitals—where most private practitioners work—the ultimate legal and moral authority lies in the hands of a board of directors composed entirely or primarily of laypersons. The board's attitude can have a major influence on the thoroughness of the peer review process.

Sometimes board members are unaware of what is going on medically within their hospital. Or, as noted in Chapter 2, hospital officials may worry that effective peer review will reduce revenues to the point where the hospital's financial status will be jeopardized. Chapter 9 contrasts peer review in two hospitals, one in which the board of directors supported a strong department head and peer review, and another in which the board offered no leadership in that area.

10. *Some cases of unnecessary surgery are difficult to detect even by conscientious peer review.* These involve situations in which the appropriateness of surgery is based on the patient's history or physical findings prior to surgery. Review of the patient's chart after the operation is not effective because doctors can record information which "passes" the review but is actually false or inaccurate. (For example, Mrs. A's gynecologist might get away with surgery by listing "excessive bleeding" as the reason even though it was not.) In such cases, only direct examination of the patient prior to surgery can provide the data necessary to judge whether surgery is needed. Protection against this type of problem can be accomplished only by means of a second opinion.

Where does the solution lie?

In my experience, the vast majority of abuses are committed by a small number of unethical doctors. Most physicians are scrupulously honest; they work hard in a demanding profession and seek the best for the patients in their care. While I would not ascribe god-like qualities to any doctors I know, I believe that most enter the profession with a high degree of compassion for and interest in their fellow humans. I cannot begin to understand the economic or personal pressures that may cause a small number to practice irresponsible medicine. Many patients can learn to recognize these practitioners and to avoid them. But the medical profession must also work hard to accomplish sincere and effective peer review.

2

UNNECESSARY SURGERY: AN OVERVIEW

Few medical issues brought to public attention have aroused the furor that surrounds the question of "unnecessary surgery." Articles on this subject have been published in medical journals as far back as 1920. But in 1970, Dr. John Bunker, a Stanford University anesthesiologist, aroused public concern by reporting that the rate of surgery was twice as high in the United States as in England.

Another leading authority on this subject is Eugene McCarthy, M.D., Professor of Public Health at Cornell University Medical Center in New York City. Dr. McCarthy pointed out that during the 30 years prior to 1971, the number of operations performed in the United States rose proportionately to our population. From 1971 to 1977, however, the number of operations increased 34 percent while the population increased only 6 percent. Part of this increase can be attributed to advances in technology, greater accessibility to medical care, the increasing wealth of our society, and expanded insurance coverage. The last item shows that people seem more willing to undergo surgery when they think someone else is paying for it.

Another factor is the demand for so-called "comfort" surgery. This is where a satisfactory medical alternative is available, but the patient thinks surgery is a more convenient or

9

comfortable approach. (The decision is usually made without sufficient regard for the risks of surgery.)

Dr. McCarthy believes that the main reason for increased surgical utilization is the large increase in the number of surgeons. Between 1971 and 1975, the supply of surgeons increased at a rate seven times faster than our general population. Studies have demonstrated that as the number of surgeons in a community increases, the number of operations tends to expand to fill their time. It has also been shown that areas with the highest number of surgeons and highest proportion of hospital beds have the highest rates of surgery. Even when hospitals are not filled to capacity, when the number of hospital beds increases, the number of hospital admissions tends to increase. These are medical versions of "Parkinson's Law"—which states that the volume of work expands to fill the amount of time available for its completion.

In 1977, with 100,000 surgeons available, there were 20 million operations. By 1982, the number of operations performed in the United States had risen to more than 34 million. During that interval the number of surgeons increased by 15 percent although the population increased by only 4 percent.

Second opinion studies

In 1972, Dr. McCarthy began to explore the issue of unnecessary surgery through large-scale studies of union workers and their dependents in the New York City area. The method he used was prospective: recommendations for surgery were evaluated before surgery was performed rather than afterward. For one group of insureds, second opinions were mandatory, and even third opinions were available upon request. In another group, they were voluntary. The consultant was not allowed to become the operating surgeon; through this mechanism it was assumed that his opinion would be unbiased. The purpose of the program was to help patients make informed decisions. But they could still have the surgery paid for if they disagreed with the consulting surgeon.

In 1976 Dr. McCarthy presented some of his findings to a subcommittee of the U.S. House of Representatives. Approximately 18 percent of the initially recommended operations were not confirmed by second opinion under the mandatory program, while 34 percent were not confirmed under the voluntary program. (Voluntary programs have higher non-confirmation rates because patients who seek voluntary second opinions have more resistance to surgery than the average patient. Mandatory programs provide a more accurate cross-section of the general population. The fact that doctors know that their opinions are being reviewed under mandatory programs also contributes to this difference in nonconfirmation rates.)

McCarthy cautioned the subcommittee that it would be improper to extrapolate his figures to estimate the total number of "surplus" operations done in the United States. He stated that his findings would not necessarily apply to all geographical areas, and more important, that it was too early to tell what proportion of individuals with nonconfirmatory second opinions would need surgery later. But by 1979, after following nonconfirmed patients for two more years, he reported that 14 percent of the recommended elective surgery he had investigated was "surplus or unnecessary."

Over the years, many articles have reported the results of second opinion programs which found high rates of nonconfirmation. Critics of these reports would then argue that these opinions must be evaluated within a longer time framework because many nonconfirmed patients will become worse and require surgery at a later date. Critics also claim that the overall (medical plus surgical) cost of treating these patients will be higher in the long run as a result of deferring their surgery.

Dr. McCarthy's data do not support either of these beliefs. After one year, 78 percent of those receiving a negative second opinion had still not had surgery. Of these, 64 percent had received no medical therapy either. Even among patients whose need for surgery was confirmed, 25 percent had elected not to go through with the procedure—and about half of this group had had no medical treatment.

It is well known that under voluntary programs, few people ask for second opinions—a fact that critics of second opinion programs are quick to point out. But Dr. McCarthy reported that patients were grateful for the mandatory feature because it gave them an excuse to offer to their physician. They were being "forced" to get a second opinion for the surgery he had recommended. They could say to their doctor that it wasn't being done because they were questioning his judgment. Without that requirement they felt they would not have had the nerve to ask for another opinion.

How prevalent is unnecessary surgery?

Since 1976 the claim that over 2 million unnecessary operations are done annually has received massive publicity. This figure was extrapolated from Dr. McCarthy's 1976 report (despite his cautions against doing this). Critics of the subcommittee's estimate, such as James H. Sammons, M.D., Executive Vice President of the American Medical Association, charged that this method involved several statistical errors. But McCarthy himself thought that 2 million was a reasonable guess in 1976. I believe that the number has increased since that time.

A number of investigators have published articles in medical journals claiming that the incidence of unnecessary surgery is much lower. For example, in 1977, Drs. Emerson and Creedin reported in the *N.Y. State Journal of Medicine* on a retrospective (after the fact) study of hysterectomies where they found less than 1 percent were unjustified. The problem with retrospective studies—as explained below and in other chapters of this book—is that some forms of unnecessary surgery cannot be identified by reading charts. They can be detected only by examining patients before surgery.

Moreover, Dr. McCarthy found that once his second opinion program was instituted, there was an 8 to 9 percent drop in the number of cases being *recommended* by the initial examining surgeon. In Saskatchewan, Canada, the rate of hysterectomies dropped 60 percent over a 4-year period after retrospective case review was begun! Dr. McCarthy calls this phenomenon the "sentinel effect." The fact that someone is watching functions as a beacon. Some doctors who tend to make blatant recommendations suddenly become more cautious. I saw this take place during my own research at a New York hospital reported later in this book. The existence of the sentinel effect is additional evidence that unnecessary surgery is a real problem. Other prospective studies have demonstrated this effect, and have also found nonconfirmation rates close to those of Dr. McCarthy.

So, although it may be impossible to measure the actual number of unnecessary operations in this country, it is clear that they are being performed in significant numbers. The goal of this book is to explore *why*—and what can be done to prevent it.

Peer review

Peer review is a method designed to achieve high standards by having group members evaluate each other's work. It is based on the assumption that voluntary self-policing is more effective than a process directed by outsiders— particularly if the outsiders lack expert training. In theory this is logical because outsiders seldom possess the expertise needed for proper evaluation. And indeed, when enough individuals are committed to such programs, great benefits accrue to all who deal with the group—in medicine, to doctors, patients and third-party payers. However, where the peer review process is not given sufficient priority, it can be ineffective or even become a sham.

The major force promoting high standards in hospitals is the Joint Commission on Accreditation of Hospitals (JCAH), sponsored by the American College of Physicians, the American College of Surgeons, the American Hospital Association and the American Medical Association. This organization sets standards, then inspects hospitals periodically to see whether the standards are being met. JCAH has enormous clout because unaccredited hospitals cannot receive direct payment for their services from Blue Cross, Medicare and Medicaid. Nor can a hospital maintain a recognized residency training program without JCAH approval.

JCAH guidelines cover virtually every aspect of hospital function, including drug utilization, medical record-keeping, blood and antibiotic usage, and infection control and bed utilization. The guidelines for peer review are excellent and quite clear: each hospital must have tissue, audit and utilization review committees.

The tissue committee is set up to review surgical specimens, pre- and postoperative diagnoses, and indications for surgery, to see whether any discrepancy exists among the findings. For example, if a surgeon were to diagnose a uterus as "grapefruit-sized with large fibroid tumors" but the uterus actually is normal and has no tumors, a discrepancy would obviously exist. Audit and utilization committees are concerned with quality of care and appropriateness of admissions.

Peer review in obstetrical and gynecological cases has an inherent problem. As discussed later in this book, some of the conditions for which surgery may be needed do not involve abnormal tissue. For example, when a uterus is removed because it has prolapsed (fallen down) too far into the vagina, the appropriateness of the surgery depends upon the extent of the prolapse or the patient's symptoms. The uterus itself will be structurally normal. Nor is abnormal tissue expected when babies are delivered by cesarean section or in the majority of cases involving breast biopsies or D&Cs. In cases of this type, the review committee's judgment must be based on the history and physical findings recorded in the chart to see whether the agreed-upon standards have been met. When a doctor writes the "correct" words, the chart will "pass" whether the words are true or not.

Medical apathy

Despite these limitations, it is clear that conscientious peer review programs can detect enough abuses to identify incompetent or dishonest practitioners. But many hospitals don't make the necessary effort. (Remember, too, that not all hospitals are accredited, and that not all hospitals engage in peer review.) The quality of the review process depends upon the percentage of cases reviewed, the care with which this is done, and the manner in which substandard practices are handled. In theory, if a practitioner is found to have a pattern of poor practice, steps should be taken to correct this problem. If no improvement is shown, the practitioner's hospital privileges can be restricted or even terminated. In practice, however, many hospitals are not doing this effectively or simply don't do it at all.

In most medical communities, there is a small group of physicians who practice substandard medicine and an even smaller group who are outright unethical. These doctors can be responsible for a significant amount of unnecessary surgery. However, the way things actually work, physicians are almost never chastised for undertaking unnecessary procedures. They get into difficulty only if they do their work poorly. The capable or even super-capable technician is almost always allowed to operate at will.

Even though many cases of unnecessary surgery can evade detection by peer review committees, some cases cannot. Moreover, gynecologists engaged in unethical practices cannot completely hide them from their colleagues. Nurses, anesthetists and resident physicians who observe unnecessary surgery may detect something wrong. Patients who seek second opinions may broadcast enough information to indicate that some doctors are engaged in improper practices. Although any one piece of data should be viewed cautiously, over a period of time it is possible to become reasonably certain how one's colleagues conduct their practices.

But even when the evidence is clear, ethical doctors are reluctant to take action against their dishonest colleagues. Although there are many more ethical than unethical physicians, somehow the minority survives. The reasons are numerous. Some doctors are afraid of controversy or of being sued by a chastised physician. Some are apathetic and don't wish to "rock the boat." Some are part of an "old boy" network even though they may be offended by the actions of a fellow physician. Should a major offender be the chief of the department or a doctor with a very high rate of admissions, the situation is even more complicated.

Another reason doctors choose not to take action against the bad apples in their midst is the fear that open criticism of medicine will cause some other force such as the government to come in to clean up the mess. On the contrary, I believe that *by allowing widespread abuses to continue, the profession opens itself to outside interference.* If doctors refuse to take action against the unethical practitioners among them, outside agencies will be more apt to take control of medicine. Doctors who choose not to act may thus create the very monster they fear the most.

It is also a harsh truth of our times that hospitals must maintain an adequate census of patients in order to remain in business. In communities with surplus hospital beds, effective peer review programs that result in fewer admissions and shorter hospital stays might lower a hospital's census to the point where its financial status will be jeopardized—a problem that would concern hospital administrators as well as physicians on the hospital staff. Also, when doctors doing the largest amount of unethical surgery happen to have the biggest practices, administrators may be afraid that disciplinary action may lead to the loss of large numbers of hospital admissions and fees.

A hospital's wish to fill its beds is not necessarily corrupt or immoral. Most hospitals are non-profit institutions whose goal is to provide the best health care within the framework of their economic stability. They must be concerned with keeping the hospital "in the black"—and that means an adequate patient census. Hospitals have a dual responsibility—to continue their existence through fiscal responsibility and to ensure that high-quality medicine is practiced within their walls. But sometimes financial pressure will cause a hospital administration to look the other way when peer review is not being conducted effectively.

Not long ago, I attended a hospital meeting where a doctor suggested that his colleagues agree to do second opinions for an insurance program with an understanding among themselves that they would always endorse the .original doctor's recommendation for surgery. Although no one took him seriously, he actually wasn't kidding.

Can women be protected?

No one honestly doubts that the great majority of surgery done is necessary and would be necessary in the eyes of any other consulting physician. It is clear that peer review is conducted effectively at some hospitals. But it is also clear that women who place blind trust in their doctors do themselves a great disservice.

Intelligent consumers should take an active role in understanding their health problems, in seeking second opinions, and in pressing for effective peer review at the hospitals in their community. This book outlines the criteria for most of the common female operations, tells where abuses are most likely to occur, and suggests how to avoid them.

3

A D&C IS NOT "MINOR" SURGERY

In all of gynecology there is no procedure less under-stood by patients than dilatation and curettage—the ubiquitous "D&C." Though doctors at times affectionately call the procedure a "dusting and cleaning," a more accurate name might be Dollars and Cents.

The D&C is a relatively simple operation. In this procedure—the second most frequently performed opera-tion throughout the United States—the lining of the uterus is scraped off (curetted) after the opening to the uterus has been stretched (dilated).

The D&C often has great value, for it allows the physi-cian to examine the contents and lining of the uterus with relative ease. Endometrial carcinoma is a malignancy of the uterine lining. Because the uterus shows changes early in the disease process, the D&C can be a powerful tool in the detection and effective treatment of uterine cancer. The excellent results now possible in the treat-ment of this disease were achieved as a result of properly performed D&Cs.

Sound reasons for doing a D&C include post-menopausal bleeding, abnormal premenopausal bleed-ing, polyps, miscarriages and a number of less common disorders. Government studies now indicate that almost one *million* D&Cs are performed each year in this country. There is no question that many of these operations are performed for perfectly valid reasons. But it is also clear that many are performed for questionable reasons— especially in young women.

Why patients are vulnerable

Most patients—and doctors too—consider the D&C so minor that few even question its appropriateness. The fact that it is a relatively minor procedure encourages its abuse. Consider the following two cases.

• Ms. B, a 24-year-old court reporter, consulted a gynecologist because she was having heavy periods. Her pelvic examination was normal. When the doctor suggested a D&C to "find out what is going on inside," Ms. B thought that seemed logical.

• Mrs. C was a 50-year-old postmenopausal woman who had been taking estrogen with the hope of preventing osteoporosis and other changes of aging. During her annual checkup she reported an episode of vaginal bleeding. Her pelvic examination was also normal. When the gynecologist advised an immediate D&C "to rule out the possibility of cancer," Mrs. C readily agreed to have the operation.

What's wrong here? In neither case did the doctor say anything about the *risks* of surgery and anesthesia. Nor did he reveal the fact that safer, more conservative approaches were available. Abnormal menstrual bleeding in young women, commonly the result of stress, can often be relieved by resolving the stress. If this approach is unsuccessful, the next step is hormonal therapy, not a D&C. And, as discussed later in this chapter, bleeding in postmenopausal women who are taking hormones is considerably more likely to be caused by the hormones than by cancer. In Mrs. C's case, stopping of the hormone, endometrial biopsy, and several months of "watchful waiting" was the simplest, safest and most prudent course of action. In occasional patients who cannot undergo endometrial biopsy because their cervix is too tightly closed, a D&C may have to be done, but Mrs. C did not have this problem.

Cases even occur where patients advised to have an unnecessary D&C feel fortunate to be under the care of a gynecologist who does not insist upon an immediate (and much more serious) surgical procedure of hysterectomy.

Why doctors are vulnerable

One could argue that the great value of the D&C as a *diagnostic* tool is a factor in the substantial abuses which are taking place. But there is no question that far too many D&Cs are performed by doctors who are well aware that other less costly forms of *treatment* would suffice. An even larger number of D&Cs are performed by physicians who convince themselves that surgery is needed—a rationalization often colored by financial considerations. Withstanding the temptation to operate—counseling a patient to follow a conservative, non-surgical course—costs the doctor money. (The surgical fee for a D&C is probably at least five times the fee for office management.) It may also cost him a patient, for in many instances the woman wishes a faster and more definitive answer to her problem and goes elsewhere to find it.

In too many cases the D&C is performed not to rule out disease or to correct some underlying problem, but for reasons that relate mainly to ignorance or greed. In my opinion, because it is easily done, and because the indications for the procedure are not clear-cut or definitive, far too many D&Cs are performed needlessly. One need only look at the medical histories of large numbers of women to comprehend the prevalence of this operation. Most women have had a D&C at some time in their lives—and many have had several. Even more significant is the fact that a large number of women had D&Cs while in their teens or early twenties, ages when the procedure is indicated only in the narrowest of circumstances.

Difficulty of peer review

To compound the potential of the D&C for abuse, there is no way to look back and determine with certainty whether the procedure was medically justifiable. Regardless of the results of pathology reports, hospital tissue committees will accept a doctor's statement on the chart that a D&C was performed for any of several reasons.

Medical restraint is weakened as well by lack of peer pressure. Using chart and tissue review alone, no one in the specialty can distinguish with certainty those D&Cs which were definitely indicated from those which were done for reasons other than good medicine. As noted in Chapter 2, blatant instances of unnecessary surgery are supposed to be picked up by hospital committees which oversee such operations at most institutions. Tissue committee members meet at regular intervals to review the pathology reports of tissue removed at operations. But because the D&C is usually done to rule out serious pathology, it is expected that most of the tissue reports will be negative; that is, the tissue removed at operation will be found to be normal.

For all of these reasons, the D&C has literally become a blank check for the unscrupulous practitioner.

Minor surgery?

During my many years of serving on tissue and utilization committees at various institutions I have never known a single D&C to be challenged as inappropriate for a patient's condition. It is equally interesting to observe that my review of the recent gynecologic literature found no important journal articles concerned with the subject of unnecessary D&Cs.

Physicians might tell you that the reason for this apparent neglect of the subject derives from the fact that it is a "minor" operation. Others warming to the subject will add that it is a definitive form of treatment that supplies immediate diagnosis, and most important, that it has relatively few complications.

But it is vitally important to note that *there is no such thing as "minor surgery" for patients who receive general anesthesia.* Any human being who does so faces some risks—ranging in severity from the mild discomfort of nausea to the possibility of cardiac arrest and death. For that reason—and for others having to do with soaring medical costs, overutilization of hospital beds and operating room facilities, and allocation of scarce medical personnel—no surgical procedure should ever be done when there is a safer, more economical, nonsurgical alternative. And in the specific instance of the D&C, there are several such alternatives. To clarify why this is so, let's look briefly at the workings of the female body.

The female hormonal system

The hormonal function of the female reproductive system is centered in the ovaries, two small glands which are controlled mainly by two structures at the base of the brain, the pituitary gland and the hypothalamus. When the ovaries are functioning properly, a rather complicated interaction among the hypothalamus, pituitary and ovary allows hormones from each of these structures to be released in varying amounts within the framework of a self-regulating pattern. The adrenal and thyroid glands also affect ovarian function but are not relevant to this discussion.

The normal ovary creates a cyclic hormonal pattern and releases an egg about once a month. For this to happen, it is necessary for the other glands to function properly. But the actions of the pituitary and hypothalamus are affected by a number of outside stimuli. These glands react markedly to weight gain, weight loss, stress and strain, significant blood loss, travel, emotional upset and numerous other transient phenomena.

When a women below the age of 40 develops some type of menstrual irregularity, such as bleeding in mid-cycle or prolonged and/or profuse menstrual flow, there are several possible causes. The bleeding can be caused by fibroids, polyps, or even malignancy, but *the most likely problem by far is hormonal: "dysfunctional uterine bleeding."* That diagnosis refers to some abnormality in the delicate hormonal balance of the pituitary, hypothalamus and ovaries. Rational medical care depends on understanding this basic concept.

Surgical vs. nonsurgical treatment

In women below 40, often the best treatment is doing nothing but watchful waiting. Again and again in my practice I have observed young women whose heavy or irregular menses correct themselves once the stress in their lives is resolved. Sometimes just knowing that no serious physical problem exists is enough to reassure the patient; and her periods revert to normal without further medical intervention.

If dysfunctional uterine bleeding persists, the doctor can rightfully conclude that some form of treatment is needed. But even then, several measures should be tried before surgery is contemplated. Since menstrual flow and other reproductive functions are governed by the balance of female hormones, the most logical approach is to see whether restoring hormonal balance solves the problem.

Dysfunctional bleeding is the body's defective attempt to shed the lining of the uterus—the endometrium—in the course of menstruation. Years ago, surgery in the form of a D&C was the only way to remove the old uterine lining and allow the patient's natural hormones to create a fresh lining that would shed more regularly in the course of monthly flow. Today we know that judicious use of hormonal therapy will often achieve the same result without surgery. The hormones build a lining in the uterus, and when they are stopped, the lining sheds. In spite of this advance, however, many gynecologists persist in using the old treatment. There are legitimate instances when a D&C is needed by a young woman whose bleeding cannot be controlled by medical means. But these occasions should be few and very far between.

Dr. Robert Greenblatt, Professor Emeritus of Endocrinology at the Medical College of Georgia, is one of the world's foremost experts in the field of gynecologic endocrinology. His writings, which span many decades of experience and relate to substantial numbers of patients, outline a rational treatment regimen for dysfunctional bleeding. For menstruating women, Dr. Greenblatt recommends hormonal rather than surgical treatment for almost all cases of dysfunctional bleeding. His regimen includes treatment with the female hormone, progesterone, in specifically defined doses, and performing an endometrial biopsy.

In this simple office procedure, the physician inserts a narrow instrument through the cervical opening and scrapes a small amount of tissue from the lining of the uterus. The material is examined carefully in the laboratory and any suspicious findings are followed by a D&C and any other necessary surgical exploration. For the vast number of women whose biopsies are normal, no further surgical measures are needed. In fact, Dr. Greenblatt stated recently that he had not performed a D&C for dysfunctional uterine bleeding in a premenopausal woman in more than 10 years! On the other hand, menopausal women who have any bleeding at all are at much greater risk and may well need a D&C.

What about women in their forties who are approaching menopause? Menstrual irregularities are not uncommon at this time. If periods become more widely spaced, nothing need be done. If periods are heavier but regularly spaced, or if bleeding occurs between periods, an endometrial biopsy may be advisable. If bleeding persists between periods, a D&C may be necessary even in the face of an endometrial biopsy.

Endometrial biopsy is simpler and safer than the D&C because it does not require stretching of the cervical opening or the use of anesthesia. The usual fee for an endometrial biopsy is about $50, while the physicians usually collect $350 or more for the average D&C! And the two procedures are almost equally effective as a screening device to rule out the presence of underlying malignancy.

Cervical polyps

Several other conditions can underlie repeated uterine bleeding in premenopausal women. One of these, cervical polyps, small and almost always benign, can cause abnormally heavy or irregular menstrual flow. These growths can easily be seen on examination of the cervix and can usually be removed in a simple office procedure that takes no more than a few minutes. But even here, the opportunity for abuse is present. I often see patients admitted to the hospital for polypectomies which could have been performed at far less cost in the office.

The polyps that occur on the cervix are of two varieties, stalked or flat (sessile). If stalked polyps are small, they can be removed in an office procedure with a minimum of bleeding. Flat polyps, on the other hand, are more likely to bleed when removed.

In my opinion, hospital-based surgery is advisable only when a danger of excessive bleeding exists. One centimeter (slightly more than ⅓-inch) is a reasonable limit for polyp removal in an office. Polyps larger than this, and sessile polyps, are less common and probably can be removed more safely in a hospital or outpatient surgical unit.

A patient really has no way to evaluate whether the procedure should or should not be done in the office. Her only recourse is to request a second opinion if removal outside of the office is suggested. Adequate hospital peer review could easily detect any physician who repeatedly operates on patients who might be handled in a much simpler and less risky manner.

Bleeding with an IUD

Some D&Cs are performed for the purpose of removing an intrauterine device (IUD). If patients using this form of contraception experience abnormally heavy periods, the physician may correctly elect to remove the IUD and wait several months to see if the excessive bleeding subsides. Here, too, opportunities for abuse are present. Physicians can claim that they are unable to remove the IUD in the office setting or that the bleeding might be caused by something other than the IUD. However, excellent instruments are available to handle most of the infrequent problems of difficult removal, and the bleeding is almost certainly caused by the IUD.

Here are the typical expenses involved in a D&C performed in a hospital to remove an IUD:

Overnight stay in a semi-private room	$ 140
Routine tests required by hospital	60
Operating room	300
Anesthesia	175
Doctor's fee	350
Total	$1,025

If the IUD were removed in an outpatient surgical unit, the cost would be about $100 less. Removal in a doctor's office can be done for the price of a routine office visit, usually $20 to $25! Even if the doctor did an endometrial biopsy as a precautionary measure during the same visit, the total charges, including examination of the tissue at the pathology laboratory, should still not exceed $100.

Postmenopausal bleeding

The onset of uterine bleeding in older women who have stopped menstruating is quite another matter. Spontaneous bleeding or spotting in a postmenopausal woman is a matter for some concern. Every gynecologist is aware of the importance of pinning down the cause of such bleeding.

Many cases of postmenopausal bleeding occur in women who are taking an estrogenic hormone to relieve the symptoms associated with menopause. In such cases, the rational medical approach is to stop the hormone, get an endometrial biopsy, and observe the patient closely to see whether the bleeding stops. But even in this relatively straightforward situation, a great many unnecessary D&Cs are being done. Indeed, the controversy surrounding the use of estrogens in postmenopausal women compounds the entire issue of appropriate treatment. In the last several years, a great deal has been written about the use of hormones to treat menopausal symptoms, because a small increase in the rate of uterine malignancy has been observed in women who have taken hormonal drugs over a long period of time. The risk is not great. Only a few years ago, the continued use of hormones was vigorously touted as a way of remaining forever young, forever female. The scientific truth about postmenopausal hormonal therapy lies somewhere between these two extremes.

A considerable amount of research indicates that judiciously used hormones can have great value both in alleviating the symptoms of menopause and preventing some of the conditions associated with aging in women. Although it is generally accepted that estrogenic therapy may cause a small increase in the malignancy rate, some of that increase may be caused by *improper* or *excessive* use of these hormones. (Continuous estrogen treatment without a monthly break is bad practice.) Overall, the great majority of patients treated with the *smallest effective dose* of female hormones will not develop cancer or unpleasant side effects, and a number of advantages will result from their use.

Although malignancy is rare, postmenopausal bleeding caused by the use of hormones is fairly common. Thus doctors who prescribe hormonal therapy should be aware that a significant percentage of recipients will bleed. They should also be willing to take the time to explain to the patient that vaginal bleeding may occur. Physicians who are not fully aware of these side effects—or who choose to disregard the fact that their therapy can underlie unusual bleeding—may rush to perform what is usually an unnecessary D&C rather than an endometrial biopsy. Physicians of this bent try to justify the surgery by explaining that it is needed to rule out cancer as the underlying cause of the postmenopausal bleeding.

The far more rational treatment plan would be to stop administering the hormones for a few months. Endometrial biopsy should also be performed during this time to look for an underlying malignancy. If the bleeding stops, it is safe to infer that hormonal therapy caused the problem. At some later date, if the patient's symptoms warrant, hormones can be restarted at a lower dosage and the patient observed again for adverse side effects.

Hormonal treatment can be made safer by adding progesterone to the estrogen therapy. When this is done in menopausal women who have already had a hysterectomy, there are almost never any side effects. However, in menopausal patients who have an intact uterus, the use of both hormones will cause them to undergo regular menstruation. Although the combined hormonal treatment decreases the slight risk of using estrogen therapy alone, most patients don't wish to continue menstrual cycles indefinitely.

Endometrial biopsy, which obtains a small sample of the uterine lining, is not as definitive as a D&C for the purpose of ruling out endometrial cancer. However, the chance that an early malignancy will be missed is extremely unlikely. If bleeding occurs after the hormones have been stopped, a D&C should definitely be performed.

Patient pressure

The physician's rationalization for doing an immediate D&C is often fueled by the patient's wish for an immediate and definitive solution. For the physician, an immediate D&C saves the time required to reassure the patient, to supply sufficient background and understanding of the problem, and then to persuade her that it is in her best interest to try other therapies before going to surgery.

Recently I met a patient in her early thirties who had been treated quite correctly with hormonal therapy for dysfunctional bleeding. The treatment process can be a slow one, with trial-and-error needed to find the most effective hormonal dose. Becoming impatient, she went to another gynecologist—who promptly recommended hysterectomy. Relieved that the second doctor had advised her to "have the damn thing out," the patient did not realize that she had undergone a hysterectomy when even a D&C was probably unnecessary!

Many women are quite pleased with the thought that hysterectomy means no more menstrual periods. This makes them very vulnerable to unnecessary surgery. Those who are unaware of the risks are even more vulnerable. As noted in Chapter 4, the complications of hysterectomy can be devastating. Hysterectomy is worth the risk only when there is a valid medical reason to do it.

I often see patients seeking a second opinion after being told by another physician, following even a single abnormal bleeding episode, that a D&C must be done immediately. This kind of irrational medical advice is offered far too frequently by gynecologists who really ought to know better. In this connection, Dr. Greenblatt has stated that there is an inverse ratio between a doctor's knowledge of female endocrinology and the number of D&Cs he will perform: the less he knows, the more D&Cs he does!

Complications of D&C

With only limited knowledge of the possible complications, an operation described as "simple" sounds logical to the patient, *but it isn't*. In the cold, impersonal terms of medicine, the overall complication rate of D&Cs has been found by different surveys to be from 0.63 to 1.7 percent. These figures are only for D&Cs unrelated to pregnancy; the complication rates of the procedure done following miscarriage or incomplete abortion are significantly higher. These figures reflect only immediate or short-term complications that arise at the time of surgery or shortly thereafter. Late complications resulting from damage to the cervix probably increase the figures somewhat, but are unreported to date.

What are the risks? We have already noted the risk associated with anesthesia. In addition, several complications are specific to the D&C:

• *Perforation* of the wall of the uterus is not rare. The uterus is an internal organ that must be explored from an external opening. Thus the operating field is necessarily limited, and the surgeon cannot view the site of the surgery, the body of the uterus itself. The operation is risky because the instruments used to perform the procedure—cervical dilators to enlarge the opening and curettes to spoon out the contents—are sharp and relatively pointed. Women who subsequently undergo abdominal surgery are sometimes found to have uterine scars indicating that an unrecognized perforation had taken place. Although perforation may not cause major aftereffects, any accidental entry into the abdominal cavity is a potentially serious event. Infection, internal bleeding, and damage to the bladder and intestine can occur.

• *Excessive bleeding* is another hazard of the D&C. When bleeding cannot be controlled by any other means, an emergency hysterectomy must be performed. Though rare, in a woman who has not fulfilled her reproductive desires, this is an especially unfortunate consequence of this "minor" surgery.

• *Infection* is a risk of any invasive procedure. In young women, infection can damage the Fallopian tubes which are critical for pregnancy and childbearing. Some experts believe that the tubal damage resulting from infection secondary to the performance of D&Cs is second only to that caused by gonorrhea.

• *Scarring* of the uterine lining, an infrequently occurring problem known as Asherman's syndrome, is another result of repeated or overly vigorous D&Cs.

Many of these complications of D&C are most critical to younger women, in whom the operation should almost never be performed in the first place! Do you still think that a D&C should be considered "minor" surgery?

An illustrative case

A 28-year-old woman who was having intercourse without using contraception came to my office worried that she couldn't become pregnant. Her fears were based on her past history. She had been treated by the same gynecologist for the past eight years for irregular menstrual cycles and occasional lower abdominal discomfort. During that period, she had been hospitalized nine times for surgery. Three abdominal operations had been done for abdominal pain. She was told the first time that she'd had a "cyst," and the other times that the pain had been caused by adhesions. On six occasions, when she had bleeding problems, a D&C was done. No attempt was ever made to use hormones to correct the bleeding problem! The woman's fear that surgery could have affected her fertility was obviously well founded. Do you think her operations were all necessary?

Sentinel effect

Several years ago, I attempted to pin down the number of D&Cs performed in a community hospital for what I consider questionable reasons. As director of its Ob-Gyn department, I had noted a steady rise in the number of D&Cs done at the hospital. I could imagine no medical reason for this and wondered why it was happening. I had also become interested in the "sentinel effect," a concept described by Dr. Eugene McCarthy in the 1970s in numerous publications as well as in his testimony before a U.S. House subcommittee studying the issue of unnecessary surgery. Dr. McCarthy, an eminent public health professor at Cornell University Medical Center, suggested that when surgeons know that their records will be reviewed, they do significantly fewer questionable operations.

For these reasons, I decided to conduct an evaluation more sophisticated than that of the hospital utilization review and tissue committees. My first step was to inspect hospital records to see how many D&Cs were done for the following reasons:

- the onset of uterine bleeding in women receiving hormones
- removal of small cervical polyps
- bleeding while an IUD remained in place
- removal of IUD's.

Despite my official staff position, I can assure you that this information was not simple to obtain! Considerable effort was needed to persuade the hospital administrator that the project should be allowed in the interest of possibly improving medical care. The administrator expressed concern about the legitimate right of patients to confidentiality of medical records. But I suspect that the real reason related to the hospital's need to fill its beds.

My survey had two parts. In the first part, I collected and tabulated data on all D&Cs done for reasons other than those related to pregnancy. The initial series excluded all those performed for termination of pregnancy, to control abnormal bleeding following delivery, and those done following miscarriage. My data covered the surgical activities of some 20 gynecologists working over a 6-month period.

Part two collected the same type of data over a subsequent 6-month period. During this time, the physicians were aware that their charts were being closely monitored. Analysis of the data revealed some remarkable information. During the second six months, the number of D&Cs performed decreased by 27 percent, from 297 to 218.

Three large private gynecological groups were operating at the time of my study. Table 3:1 shows how the operative rate went down for each group as well as for the remainder of gynecologists.

Even more interesting were the data relating to the ages of the patients. The risks of uterine malignancy in menopausal women is considerably greater than that for women in their 20s or 30s. To evaluate these D&Cs, I looked at the number of operations done on young women where the risk of malignancy is extremely low. The initial series of 297 disclosed 11 cases of uterine cancer. The sec-

Table 3:1. Sentinel effect (shown by decrease in number of D&Cs)

Doctors	Initial Study (Doctors Unaware)	Second Study (Doctors Aware)	Percentage Change
Group A	49	27	−45%
Group B	68	53	−22%
Group C	85	59	−30%
Rest of staff	95	79	−17%
Total	297	218	−27%

ond series also contained 11 cases, but there were far fewer patients—only 218. This difference occurred because fewer patients under 50 had the operation when the doctors knew they were being observed. In the first series, 67 percent of the women were under 50 years of age and 33 percent were beyond that. In the second group, 60 percent were under 50, and 40 percent were over 50. This was an improvement, though still far from ideal. Although endometrial cancer occurs in women under the age of 50, in this series of more than 500 women, the 22 cases found were all in postmenopausal women over the age of 50.

The more appropriately cases are selected, the higher will be the percentage of cases found with malignancies. Table 3:2 shows how the percentage of malignancies rose when the doctors knew they were being observed.

One should not conclude from the preceding discussion that the only reason for performing the D&C is to identify malignancies. However, the fear that cancer may be present often serves as the bait to induce the patient to undergo surgery, especially if the information is presented in a highly sensational way. But the knowledge that endometrial cancinoma is quite rare in younger women should be sufficient to arm a well-informed patient against the entreaties of irrational medicine.

Table 3:2. Sentinel effect on percentage of D&Cs finding cancer

Doctors	Cancer rate (doctors unaware)	Cancer rate (doctors aware)	Rate of improvement
Group A	2.0%	7.4%	270%
Group B	4.4%	5.7%	30%
Group C	4.7%	5.1%	9%
Remainder of staff	3.2%	3.8%	19%

Even more interesting was the information revealed by analysis of the data on postmenopausal women whose bleeding occurred while they were taking estrogenic hormones—usually prescribed by the same physician who performed the operation. In the total survey period of one year, 16 women on estrogenic hormones had undergone a D&C without first being taken off the medication and observed to see if the uterine bleeding would stop within a reasonable period of time. Although the supposed justification for such operations is to rule out malignancy, not one of these 16 patients was found to have uterine cancer!

Now it is true that a hidden malignancy might have been uncovered in the course of one of these D&Cs. But it is equally true that a far less costly endometrial biopsy would very likely have revealed the same information. In all of these cases, merely terminating the use of hormones would have stopped the bleeding. Had it not, the patients could then have undergone a D&C.

These data support my belief that many D&Cs done in postmenopausal women are unnecessary, especially in women taking estrogenic hormones. In my survey, many of these operations appeared to be done by the doctors who use the hormones most injudiciously and, as a result, cause the greatest incidence of postmenopausal bleeding in their patients!

Equally striking are the data derived from D&Cs done to remove cervical polyps. My first survey found that 14 out of 21 were performed to remove small polyps which could have been removed in the doctor's office. After I dropped my bombshell on my colleagues by announcing that I would examine subsequent records, the "sentinel effect" took place: the second series of 16 cases included only 5 in which the polyps were small. In my opinion, the appropriate number should be close to zero!

The same pattern was apparent when I examined records pertaining to D&Cs done for the removal of IUDs. The first survey found that 12 patients underwent the operation for bleeding associated with an in-place IUD. In the second survey, the number dropped to six, once again demonstrating the sentinel effect. Table 3:3 summarizes some of these findings.

Table 3:3. Sentinel effect on D&C

Stated reason for operations	Initial study (doctors unaware)	Follow-up study (doctors aware)
Number of D&Cs	297	218
Incidence of malignancy	3.7%	5.0%
Incidence of malignancy in patients under age 50	0.0%	0.0%
Percentage of D&Cs in patients under age 50	66.7%	60.0%
Percentage of D&Cs for undersized polyps	66.7%	31.3%
D&Cs for IUD removal	12	6
Probable percentage of inappropriate D&Cs	over 35%	25%

D&Cs related to pregnancy

Records were also examined involving pregnancy-related D&Cs. These include a large number done at the time of the miscarriage, a clouded area because the scientific literature contains no accurate information on how often it is really necessary to do a D&C in that circumstance. Although there are many instances in which the bleeding following miscarriage can be controlled only by curettage, it is also true that it need not be done in every instance of incomplete abortion. In many cases, especially miscarriages of less than six weeks' gestation (before a second period is missed), most of the tissue will have been passed, or if the patient is properly informed and willing to wait, will be passed through light bleeding in the weeks following miscarriage or in the course of the next menstrual period.

But again, this requires considerable time on the part of the physician—he must explain the options and counsel the patient that she may still have to undergo surgery if the bleeding increases. The financial difference to the physician is considerable. A D&C performed on a patient for a miscarriage is routinely billed at approximately $350. If the patient is allowed to pass it by herself, the total cost may be no more than a routine office visit.

A patient recently told me of her experience following miscarriage in the 6th week of pregnancy. While in the emergency room she overheard a resident say that there was no reason for her to have a D&C because most of the tissue had been passed and the bleeding was minimal. When her physician arrived, he strongly recommended surgery and she was able to avoid an unnecessary D&C only by signing herself out of the hospital. If this patient had not accidentally acquired the information she needed to make a rational decision, she would have undergone a totally unneeded operation. My research indicates that many D&Cs done in these circumstances are indeed unnecessary.

In pregnancy-related cases as well as in non-pregnancy cases, my study observed the sentinel effect: when aware that they are being watched, doctors perform fewer D&Cs for reasons that are marginal. The corollary is that physicians as a group provide better care when there is better policing. The reason for this is that most abuses are the work of a small number of physicians. In the series of operations I studied, I was able to observe the significant effect of a small group of physicians who practice reckless, irrational medicine. Do you think that most hospitals police this problem effectively?

The results of my initial survey, presented to a meeting of the hospital's gynecologic staff were greeted with hostility, anger and a considerable amount of bad feeling. My colleagues demanded to know what right I had to review their work. It was a long time before these feelings subsided.

Whose physician is the unethical one?

My initial computation found that one group of physicians was performing three to five times as many D&Cs to discover the same number of malignancies as the other physicians in that hospital. If all the other gynecologists in an institution find malignancies in 3½ to 5 percent of cases, should we accept and tolerate a rate of 2 percent? That particular group of physicians was doing almost 20 percent of all D&Cs performed—a clearcut example of hazardous medicine.

My study found that for every physician or group, whether data in the first series seemed acceptable or not, there was an increasing rate of malignancies in the follow-up data. In one group of doctors, the increase was almost *four* times as great in the follow-up series than had been found in the earlier data. The sentinel effect was working. Other research projects have found similar results.

Should consumers accept the fact that 20 percent of patients admitted for surgery are under the care of an unethical physician, even if most physicians are ethical? Would patients feel safe and secure if they know there is no way for them to be certain whether they are in the hands of an unethical physician because no one is controlling that doctor?

What does this all mean?

I believe that a significant number of D&Cs are performed in the costly hospital setting for conditions that can be treated in the doctor's office at far less cost and with far less risk to the patient. My belief was confirmed by observing the sentinel effect: when the physicians in my institution knew that their subsequent records would be reviewed, the number of inappropriate or questionable D&Cs dropped significantly. The main reason for this effect is that the small number of less-than-ethical physicians, who are responsible for the majority of the abuses, will provide better care when they know they are being watched.

Some unnecessary D&Cs are the result of faulty rationalization; others may be motivated by greed, or ignorance. Most important for patients to understand, however, is that like most unnecessary operations, inappropriately performed D&Cs are almost *never* picked up by the institutional forces which are supposed to be protecting the public. Tissue committees, hospital utilization committees, and even the possibility of lawsuits charging malpractice, provide little or no defense against *well-performed* procedures. A badly performed operation, or even a well-performed one in which the outcome is unexpectedly disastrous, is often the object of some kind of censure. Bad results can be noted and investigated by department chiefs, hospital administrators and most often, by patients themselves—but well-performed, unnecessary D&Cs will almost never be questioned.

Pressure from an informed public is needed to change this situation.

4

WHO NEEDS A HYSTERECTOMY?

Mrs. D saw her gynecologist for a "routine" pelvic examination. She had no symptoms but had come for her 6-month checkup. She was now 38 years old. Three years ago the doctor had advised her that the risk of gynecological disease increases significantly at age 35 and that it would therefore be advisable for her to come twice a year. (As noted in Chapter 7, this type of recommendation is irresponsible.)

After examining Mrs. D's uterus, the doctor said that the small fibroid tumor he had been watching for a number of years had grown considerably, and there was now a cyst present in her left ovary. He expressed concern over the reason for this sudden change and recommended that she undergo immediate surgery—a hysterectomy with removal of her tubes and ovaries as well as her uterus. Frightened, Mrs. D sought another opinion. The consulting physician found a minimally enlarged fibroid uterus, but no increase in ovarian size, and said that surgery was obviously not needed. Fibroids are rarely associated with cancer (only about 1 in 200 cases) and do not require removal unless they become large or troublesome enough to cause symptoms.

Mrs. E, a woman in her early thirties was sent to me for

a second opinion by her insurance carrier. During her mid-twenties, her gynecologist had advised her to undergo surgery for an ovarian cyst—which she did. She later had an operation for vague lower abdominal complaints and was told that the problem was adhesions secondary to the first operation.

At the time of her visit to me, her complaint once again was vague lower abdominal pain. She told me that her doctor had ordered x-ray examinations of her gallbladder, stomach and intestines as well as an ultrasound of her lower abdomen and pelvis. These tests uncovered no abnormalities, but she was informed that the pelvic exam had revealed an ovarian cyst and that she needed a hysterectomy.

When I examined her, I felt no abnormality whatsoever. I contacted the physician directly to ascertain his findings. He told me that he had felt nothing abnormal and that the ultrasound had revealed no ovarian cyst. When I asked him what the indication for the hysterectomy would be, he responded that once the ovaries were removed there was no need to leave the uterus. (This response presupposed there was a reason to remove the ovaries.) I then asked why the ovaries had to be removed. His response was, "Maybe there is something wrong with them."

Of course I advised Mrs. E not to have surgery.

Scare tactics

The foregoing stories are not cases of medical error, but of *fraud*. The uterus is a favored target for a small number of unscrupulous doctors who deliberately use scare tactics to persuade patients to have high-priced, unneeded surgery. The approach includes statements like:

"This is something bad for you. Who knows what it will cause in the future, so it must come out!"

"Why do you need or want your uterus? Now that you've had your children it ought to come out!"

—and worst of all—

"We can't tell when that will become malignant. It had better come out now!"

THE CANCER SCARE! It takes a well-informed patient to walk away from that one!

The fact that only a few doctors do this sort of thing is no consolation—because each of them can wind up doing a great many unnecessary operations.

Moreover, there is another problem which does not involve fraud but can be just as serious for patients: hysterectomy performed where nonsurgical treatment would be a safer and less costly—and therefore a better— alternative. The percentage of cases in which needless surgery is performed is impossible to pin down—but it is not small.

Many studies exploring the issue of unnecessary surgery have yielded data on proper indications for hysterectomy, cost-effectiveness of the surgery, risk/benefit ratios, and nonconfirmation rates of second opinions. In 1981, for example, five researchers at Stanford University reported on a study they had done for the Office of Technology Assessment of the U.S. Congress. They concluded that 30 percent of the hysterectomies in the United States were performed to sterilize the women or to prevent the occurrence of uterine or cervical cancer. After thorough analysis, they found that: 1) hysterectomy is more costly and not as safe as tubal ligation; and 2) the risk of the operation itself outweighs the possible gain in cancer prevention in healthy individuals when one considers non-fatal complications. The researchers therefore recommended that hysterectomies be used for sterilization only when an abnormal condition is present. In 1983, Blue Cross and Blue Shield of Greater New York reported the results of their second opinion program. It was a voluntary program that evaluated over 1,500 surgical cases over a 20-month period. The nonconfirmation rate for hysterectomies was 29.7 percent. About half of "nonconfirmed" patients have surgery at a later date, but the other half do not need it and can be considered "unnecessary." Similar percentages have been found in many other studies.

Who needs a hysterectomy

Over 650,000 hysterectomies are done each year in the United States. There are six basic situations in which the operation is appropriate:

    1. Cancer of the cervix, uterus, ovaries or fallopian

tubes. The diagnosis of these conditions can usually be made prior to surgery through the use of such studies as pap smears, colposcopy, cervical biopsy, endometrial biopsy, D&C, sonography, and of course, pelvic examination.

2. Diseases of the tubes and ovaries where the uterus in not primarily involved but must be removed because of its closeness to the diseased areas. One example would be a severe chronic infection of the tubes. Another would be severe endometriosis, a noncancerous condition in which tissue resembling the uterine lining grows in various parts of the pelvis.

3. Involvement of the uterus in non-gynecological diseases such as cancer of the colon or a severe infection (abscess) secondary to diverticulitis.

4. An obstetrical catastrophe such as uncontrollable bleeding after delivery, uterine rupture or massive infection.

5. Severe prolapse of the uterus. This is a condition in which the uterus has descended through the pelvis to the vaginal opening or beyond due to loss of the normal supporting tissue.

6. Some cases of fibroid tumors of the uterus. These are firm masses of fibrous tissue growing in the walls of the uterus. They are almost always noncancerous.

The decision to remove the uterus for the first four conditions listed above is usually clear-cut and noncontroversial—and involves virtually no abuse by doctors. The last two, however, are the objects of much abuse; great care must be used to determine whether surgery is needed. Let's look at these in detail.

Uterine prolapse

In mild cases of prolapse, the cervix extends part-way down the vagina; in more severe cases, the cervix can reach to the vaginal opening or even outside of it. Prolapse is almost always secondary to the effects of pregnancy and childbirth. Although many women have their uterus located considerably lower than it was before they gave birth, few of them have symptoms as a result. However, in some cases, the descent is sufficient to cause considerable discomfort in the form of backache or feelings of pressure or heaviness.

There are gynecologists, who upon finding the *slightest* drop in the uterus, will immediately tell their patient, "Your uterus must come out. If you don't have it removed now, it will get progressively worse and cause very serious problems." That simply is untrue. Many women with moderate prolapse would not even be aware of it unless a physician called it to their attention. In many such cases, further descent would not occur. Over the years, most women with uterine prolapse who have consulted me for a second opinion did not need surgery!

Patients who *do* need surgery see a doctor because they have severe discomfort from the prolapse or have major urinary symptoms of a specific type called "stress incontinence." This is a condition in which urine leaks out when the patient coughs, sneezes, laughs hard or exercises; or in severe cases, when she just walks about. However, women with urinary frequency or a constant urge to urinate, but no loss of control of urinary function, do not have stress incontinence and can usually be treated with medication and pelvic floor exercises. Some women with minimal stress incontinence can even be treated in this manner.

When surgery is needed, the usual operation is vaginal hysterectomy, a procedure in which the uterus is removed through the vaginal canal without any abdominal incision. When this operation can be performed with relative ease, it usually requires less time in the hospital and has a shorter recovery period than abdominal hysterectomy. However, the vaginal approach is not practical when the uterus is too large or when adhesions (scar tissue) of the uterus, tubes or ovaries are present. The decision concerning vaginal or abdominal approach should be individualized by the physician for each patient.

When uterine prolapse with pressure symptoms exists in an elderly woman who is a poor surgical risk, surgery can often be avoided by the use of a pessary, a device inserted into the vagina to hold up the fallen uterus and, if necessary, the vaginal walls as well. Although using a pessary for many years is not practical for younger women, for the elderly, it is frquently a blessing. Many of the women who have been quietly miserable for years with their uterus projecting from the vagina become eternally grateful when their pressure symptoms are relieved, and don't mind at all having to return every few months to have the device cleaned and reinserted.

Treatment with medication, exercise or a pessary is not highly remunerative to the physician and therefore may not be offered as a possible alternative to surgery. There is certainly no reason not to try the simpler methods of treatment before resorting to the surgical approach. Moreover, in some cases of prolapse with no urinary symptoms and no need for surgery, patients will develop major urinary problems as a result of the unnecessary operation!

Proper management of fibroids

Uterine fibroids are so common that it behooves all women to understand their significance and what to do if a doctor suggests that they be removed. When a fibroid uterus is accompanied by symptoms that cannot be corrected by other means, hysterectomy may be the proper treatment. *However, when no symptoms exist and the fibroids are discovered during a pelvic examination, the need for surgery should be very carefully evaluated.*

Patients with fibroids may seek treatment because of abnormal bleeding, pain, or urinary or bowel problems; or they may have no symptoms at all.

If *abnormal bleeding* is the presenting symptom, an endometrial biopsy or D&C should be done. If *cancer* is found, proper treatment can be started. If there is no malignancy, the treatment should vary, depending upon whether or not an irregularity is felt on the inner surface of the uterus at the time of the biopsy. If the inner surface is irregular, indicating that fibroids are projecting into the uterine lining, if bleeding persists, and if childbearing has been completed, a hysterectomy can be performed. If the lining is not irregular, the bleeding is probably caused by a hormonal disturbance that often can be controlled by hormonal treatment. If hormonal treatment is not successful and childbearing has been complete, a hysterectomy may be necessary.

If *pain* is the primary symptom, it is likely that the fibroids are of considerable size. If the pain cannot be controlled and childbearing has been completed, a hysterectomy may have to be done.

If the primary symptoms are *urinary frequency and urgency* caused by pressure of the uterus on the bladder, it may be possible to correct them with bladder exercises. *Severe constipation* caused by pressure of fibroids on the large intestine is a more difficult problem. If urinary or bowel symptoms persist and childbearing has been completed, a hysterectomy is the best treatment. However, it should be stressed that for these symptoms to occur, the uterus usually must be quite large—and this is rare. Constipation should be investigated carefully to be sure it does not have another cause.

In cases where childbearing is still desired, it may be possible to avoid surgery altogether or to perform an operation (myomectomy) which removes the fibroid but leaves the uterus, ovaries and tubes intact. When childbirth is no longer desired, myomectomy should not be performed because it is a more complicated operation than a hysterectomy.

When there are *no symptoms*, follow-up pelvic examinations should be done to see whether the uterus is enlarging. If enlargement of a fibroid uterus appears to be taking place, it should be confirmed with sonography. In those rare instances where the uterus is found to be growing rapidly, surgery should be considered because of the possibility that cancer may be present.

It is generally agreed that hysterectomy is appropriate when large fibroids are accompanied by abnormally heavy bleeding, pain or pressure that cannot be managed by nonsurgical means. The uterus in such cases is usually at least the size of a 12-week pregnancy. However, many women with fibroids that size have no symptoms whatsoever; and there is *absolutely* no reason for them to undergo such surgery! The risk of malignancy in fibroids is extremely low, and there is no evidence to demonstrate that the 12-week size fibroid is more likely to be malig-

Table 4:1. Management of Fibroids

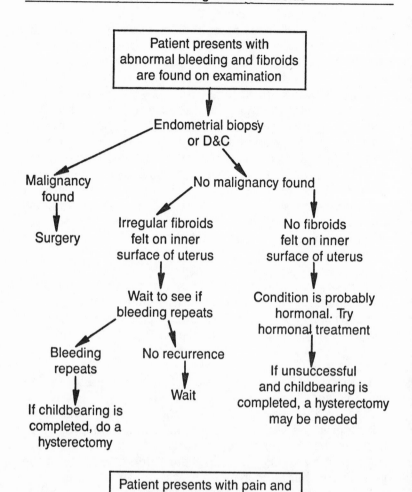

Table 4:1. Management of Fibroids (Cont.)

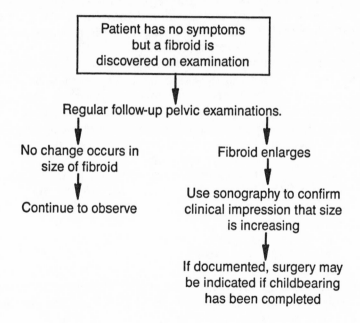

Patient has difficulty with
urination and/or bowel
movements. (Usually seen only
with large fibroids.)

Urinary symptoms may be controlled by bladder
exercise. Difficulty in having bowel movements due to
pressure is harder to help. If childbearing is completed,
then hysterectomy may be the best choice.

Patient has no symptoms
but a fibroid is
discovered on examination

Regular follow-up pelvic examinations.

No change occurs in
size of fibroid

Continue to observe

Fibroid enlarges

Use sonography to confirm
clinical impression that size
is increasing

If documented, surgery may
be indicated if childbearing
has been completed

In all cases where childbearing is still desired,
the possibility of either avoiding surgery
or having a myomectomy should be considered

nant. Moreover, many fibroids become smaller after menopause. Thus if a woman can tolerate their presence until menopause takes place, the fibroids may cease to be a problem.

Table 4:1 summarizes how the need for hysterectomy can be evaluated when fibroids are present.

Less-than-sufficient reasons

A general point of view has grown among gynecologists that a 12-week-size fibroid gives the physician-"finder" outright license to claim that patient for a hysterectomy. Whether the patient is having symptoms or not, the 12-week-size fibroid must come out!

Some doctors who make this recommendation rationalize that fibroids are abnormal and therefore should come out. They say to themselves and to their patients, "Why take chances? Let's get rid of it." Faced with this type of suggestion, many women readily agree and proceed to surgery. If no complications occur, they may be quite pleased with their care. But the fact is that about one-third of women develop fibroids and the vast majority of fibroids produce no symptoms at all! Even when symptoms occur, they can often be managed without surgery and disappear after menopause.

A small percentage of doctors involved in this process are not rationalizing but are involved in deliberate fraud. They know that surgery is not needed and simply want to raise their incomes.

Table 4:2 illustrates how doctors varied in their approach to hysterectomy at the community hospital I surveyed in 1981. The comparison is based on the fact that hysterectomies on women over age 40 are much more likely to be appropriate than those under age 40. I believe that the doctors with the lowest rates are considered the most capable and most ethical gynecologists on the hospital staff. It is a safe assumption that doctors who do most of their hysterectomies on women under 40 are practicing improperly.

A common dilemma

The majority of female patients may face the risk of

Table 4:2. Hysterectomy rates for doctors doing at least 9 hysterectomies during 1981

Doctor	No. hysterectomies	No. patients under age 40	% patients under age 40
#1	9	7	78%
#2	23	17	74%
#3	15	11	73%
#4	17	12	71%
#5	40	27	68%
#6	52	35	67%
#7	15	10	67%
#8	12	8	67%
#9	20	13	65%
#10	13	8	62%
#11	72	44	61%
#12	31	19	61%
#13	22	12	55%
#14	61	32	52%
#15	18	9	50%
#16	28	13	46%
#17	9	4	44%
#18	14	6	43%
#19	15	6	40%
#20	16	6	38%
#21	35	10	29%
#22	35	9	26%
#23	19	5	26%
#24	88	21	24%
#25	18	4	22%

unnecessary hysterectomy at some time in their lives. A woman may have a gynecologist she has used with trust, often for many years. She has a very strong feeling of loyalty to her doctor whom she has evaluated as being very fine. Her judgment is for the most part quite accurate. However, a time may arrive in her care when a health problem arises that has several possible solutions. One alternative is watchful waiting or the use of some simple medication. The other alternative is surgery.

The surgical approach has a certain appeal to patient and physician. The problem is attacked definitively. There will be an immediate answer to the question of exactly what is happening and very likely a quick solution. This approach, however, is not altogether harmless. Many women who undergo hysterectomy experience complications such as fever, bleeding, infection or pelvic pain, and one or two of every thousand die. Only the fool-hardy consider that there is any surgical procedure without risk. Patients can die or have major complications from the most minor types of surgery. In making a choice of therapy, it is critical to remember that *no surgery should be undertaken lightly.*

The usual reason for unnecessary hysterectomy is economic. Money is a driving force in most people's lives. The physician is not without the same pressures that everyone else faces. Operating an office costs more money than most people realize. The typical gynecologist must earn somewhere between $1,000 and $1,500 per week to meet office expenses. This estimate is not presented to solicit pity for the physician, for in fact, I don't know any physicians who live in poverty. Like many others who wish to earn a certain amount of money to take care of expenses and perceived personal needs and desires, physicians have the opportunity to decide how that money can be earned. Hysterectomy fees generally range from $800 to $1,500.

Is there any doubt that if a consumer's decision to buy or not in the normal marketplace (food, clothing, etc.) were determined by the seller of the commodity, the decision would be to buy? How many sellers pass up sales opportunities by telling potential customers to shop elsewhere?

If this is a cynical approach to medicine, then the cynicism is not without cause. Pause for a moment and understand the nature of the problem. The patient presents with a condition which is *properly and ethically* handled either surgically or nonsurgically. In one choice, nonsurgical, the physician gets little remuneration for his watchful waiting. The patient may be made nervous and anxious by such non-definitive care. The problem has not been solved immediately and demands a certain amount of patience from both parties involved.

What about the surgical approach? The patient may not be made adequately aware of the risks, expense, and other aspects involved with the hospitalization and loss of time. The expense factor itself may be minimized, based on the fact that insurance will be the major source of the funds. However, we should all understand that ultimately the money must come from consumers, whether through direct payment, insurance premiums, or taxes.

Considering all this, an average physician may easily rationalize the need for the surgery. He convinces himself that it is the very best thing he can do for his patient. He loses sight of the possibility that the surgery might be unnecessary. Should he decide whether surgery is a proper choice when his decision is based on a conflict of interest? I think not! Patients for whom the advice to operate was not unethical but yet was *questionable* can be found regularly in most hospitals.

For 18 years situations like these have arisen in my office. I have had to make the same decisions. I know the feeling very well. My practice and my income, like that of every other private practitioner, depends on how much work I do. I have gone through the process of treating a patient with the possible need for surgery. I know the difficulty involved in saying to myself, "Can you avoid doing this surgery you are contemplating?" When the answer is yes, and my days and weeks have been particularly devoid of work, I know that it takes all my willpower to say, "Don't have surgery now! Don't let anyone operate on you!" I am not now referring to blatantly unnecessary surgery. I refer to proper treatment that might better be replaced by proper but less remunerative nonsurgical therapy.

I have had the opportunity to provide the second opinion in a large number of cases where the patient has requested the consultation. In approximately three-fourths of those cases, I have advised against the recommended surgery and suggested medical management or a much more minor surgical procedure instead. This does not mean that 75 percent of recommended surgery is unnecessary. The percentage is probably that high because these were patients who had doubts—and rightly so, it turned out. *These were consultations sought in an environment where second opinions for possible surgery have not been encouraged.* Where second opinions regarding hysterectomy have been mandatory, a 30 percent nonconfirmation rate is commonly seen—and more than half of these patients are able to avoid the surgery.

Pitfalls in peer review

At most hospitals, any gynecologist who honestly evaluates the surgery taking place knows that unnecessary operations are being done. Sadly, from my own experiences, that is certainly true. There are some areas where peer review and the evaluation of specific physicians' actions are almost unheard of.

Remember that tissue and utilization committees make their judgments after the fact, based on medical records. Physicians are well aware of the criteria used to evaluate their charts. In cases where the uterus and other tissue removed are normal, the patient's history will usually involve a list of symptoms. The utilization review process does not attempt to determine whether the history has been recorded honestly.

The size of a fibroid uterus can be misjudged. Whether this is due to the difficulty in making such judgments or just convenient misevaluation varies from case to case. But some physicians make this type of error repeatedly. They record in their admitting physical examination the presence of a "12 to 14-week size uterus." When the organ is removed from the body, somehow it is only 6 weeks' size. *This is a considerable difference*—like that between a lemon and a grapefruit. We may think of such physicians kindly and merely consider them inept. However, physicians who make repeated "errors" of this kind may not be doing do so accidentally. Certainly, a minority of gynecologists are guilty of blatant mismeasurement, but once again, in a hospital where peer review is inadequate, they may do a great many unnecessary operations.

Vaginal hysterectomy is more prone to being done needlessly than is abdominal hysterectomy because controls are more difficult to achieve. Though it is frequently an indicated operation, the doctor can easily falsify information in the patient's chart to make the procedure appear properly chosen.

In cases of vaginal hysterectomy for prolapse, for example, the utilization committee will consider the operation justified if the patient had a prolapse of the uterus and significant symptoms along with that condition. The fact that the removed uterus is anatomically normal will not disturb the committee because this is expected in cases of uterine prolapse. The doctor didn't claim there is anything wrong with the uterus, only its position. Anyone evaluating the chart will find no abnormalities except in the history given by the physician, but that will automatically qualify the surgery as "necessary."

Thus women who wish to avoid unnecessary hysterectomy must become medically sophisticated and make use of second opinions.

5

CESAREAN SECTIONS: HOW MANY IS TOO MANY?

There is probably no area in medicine that attracts more personal interest, especially from women, than the process of childbirth. Most women believe that delivering a baby vaginally is one of the most marvelous experiences a woman can have. The possibility of having that opportunity supplanted by abdominal surgery certainly causes many pregnant women to worry: "Will I be the one to have a cesarean section—and if so, why?"

The answer to that "why" is usually quite satisfactory: when vaginal delivery is difficult or impossible, a "C-section" can make the difference between life and death or severe injury to the baby—and possibly to the mother as well. The operation is relatively simple. Under anesthesia, during which the patient may be awake or asleep, an incision is made through the layers of the abdominal wall. The uterus is then cut open and the child delivered through the opening. Most of the 45 minutes the operation typically takes is used to close the surgical incisions from the uterus outward through each layer of the abdomen.

This chapter explores the fact that many cesareans are being done for less-than-adequate reasons.

Historical background

Cesarean sections, though not called by that name, were referred to in the earliest Persian mythology. Somewhere in the vicinity of 100 A.D., the ancient Hebrews reported C-sections being performed by Theodorus, a noted physician. The Hindus as well were performing abdominal surgical deliveries. These were attempted when vaginal delivery was impossible and the alternative would have been death of both mother and child.

The name of the operation arises from Roman civilization, though its results were not nearly so successful as those reported by the Hebrews or Hindus. Contrary to popular belief, the operation did not receive its name because Julius Caesar was born by a surgical approach. At the time of his birth, cesarean sections all resulted in the death of the mother, either before or after delivery. Since letters from Caesar to his mother provide good evidence that she survived his birth, it can be deduced that she delivered vaginally. The operation's name actually arose from the law, *Lex Caesare*, which commanded that if a woman should die while pregnant, the doctor must immediately cut out the baby.

During the 16th century, 15 successful C-sections with surviving mothers were recorded. But in Paris during that same period, maternal death from infection was so frequent that the operation was barred in that city until the 17th century. During most of the 18th century, cesareans were used primarily to try to save the baby when the mother's life was considered unsalvageable. Though a few mothers survived, significant success rates were not achieved until late in the 19th century with the development of sterile surgical techniques.

Survival rates increased still further as anesthesia and blood replacement became commonplace. By the mid-1920s, the operation was an established part of obstetrical practice. Death rates had fallen sharply, but were still significant. For example, a major hospital in Detroit reported that 1 out of 200 deliveries were accomplished by C-section with a maternal death rate of 13 percent, while an English hospital reported a maternal death rate of 6.9 percent.

The discovery of antibiotics led to a dramatic improvement in the maternal survival rate during the mid-1940s. The above-noted Detroit hospital reported a C-section rate of 3 percent, with a maternal death rate of 0.8 percent, while the same English hospital reported a death rate of 1 percent. In 1944, doctors at New Haven Hospital reported 663 consecutive C-sections with 2 maternal deaths, a rate of 0.3 percent. During the same period, the Boston Lying-In Hospital had a maternal death rate of 1.3 percent and a Chicago Hospital had 2 deaths in 500 cases—0.4 percent. By 1958, when I graduated from medical school and began clinical exposure to obstetrics and gynecology, the maternal mortality rate had fallen still lower.

My first taste of hazardous medicine

Although C-sections had obviously become much safer, safety was not the only factor that influenced the decision to operate. Because almost all deliveries had to be performed vaginally, physicians developed great expertise in many complicated maneuvers for delivering problem cases by the vaginal route. There was a "macho" aspect to obstetrics that is almost hard to believe now. Perhaps it was partly due to the fact that almost all obstetricians were men. Privileged to oversee perhaps woman's most precious "gift"—the ability to carry and deliver a new life— these doctors typically did so with a sense of paternalism. They "knew" what was best for the so-called "weaker" half of society and would decide what should be done for mother and baby.

During the process of labor, it is necessary for the baby's head to descend into the pelvis before delivery can be accomplished. Anatomical landmarks at different levels of the female pelvis are used to denote points which are named "high," "mid-" and "low" pelvic positions. Generally a fetus will not descend below the high pelvic position when the baby is too large to fit through the mother's pelvis. During the days when C-section was extremely dangerous to the mother, doctors would attempt to grasp the baby high in the pelvis with forceps and pull it out. Although high forceps could injure the mother's uterus, vagina or bladder, it was still far safer for the mother than cesarean section—so much so that risks to the baby (which were considerable and included brain damage) were not a factor in the decision.

Another procedure used back then was internal podalic version. This involved turning the baby inside the uterus from a head-first position into a breech (buttocks-first) presentation before delivering it. Even if one ignores the increased risk of delivering a breech, which we are aware of today, internal podalic version is a treacherous technique. Rotation of a full-term baby in what is a relatively thin-walled container by that stage in the pregnancy, runs a terrible risk of rupturing the uterus and killing the baby (and possibly the mother as well).

By the mid-1950s, the risk of high forceps was so much greater than that of C-section that it was no longer part of rational medical practice; and internal podalic version had become obsolete, except for occasional use in delivering the second of a set of twins. But many obstetricians kept doing these procedures. Some, no doubt, preferred to stick with what they were used to. Others, caught up in their own egos, believed, "I can get that baby out vaginally—no matter what." The more difficult the delivery, the greater the challenge they felt.

It was then that I had my first exposure to hazardous medicine—one which has remained in my memory for almost 25 years. I was a young resident learning the mechanical skills which would enable me to accept all the most difficult challenges. I was being taught that, though the risks were great, the mark of my ability as an obstetrician would be whether I could perform the most difficult deliveries with the least amount of trauma to mother and baby. Unfortunately, as a result of such thinking, some babies were unnecessarily jeopardized.

Among my mentors was a senior member of the department who had developed a reputation for miraculous deeds in the delivery room. By the time I became a resident, internal podalic version was no longer considered appropriate for delivering a single infant. My teacher, for whom I had the greatest respect, decided one day in the midst of a normal, simple vaginal delivery that it was time for me to learn this difficult and dangerous maneuver. He wanted me to try the technique so that when the day came that I had to use it, I would have the necessary experience. I recall how proud I was when the deed was done—but not for long.

Within a short time, word of what had occurred in the delivery room that day got back to the head of the department. In no time, both I and the senior obstetrician, who was second in command only to the director, were called in to his office. What followed was directed mainly at my teacher. The director warned him that should he ever "pull such a stunt again"—placing his ego ahead of the safety and welfare of a mother and child—he would be stripped of his position. The director then said to me, a rather scared young man, that he wanted me to learn a lesson. Regardless of the outcome, I had unnecessarily taken two lives into my hands.

What had prompted my mentor to lead me down such a dangerous path? Two factors were probably involved. In those days it was important to achieve great dexterity in vaginal deliveries, since obstetricians considered themselves less than adequate if their C-section rate was over 3 or 4 percent. He wanted me to leave my training as manually skilled as he considered himself. He probably also had an underlying desire to demonstrate his prowess.

From those days until the present, the circumstances under which a C-section is safer for mother and child than a vaginal delivery have gradually become clearer. At the same time, the rate of cesarean sections has risen.

Primary vs. repeat C-sections

To evaluate C-section statistics, it is necessary to understand the difference between primary and repeat C-sections. Primary cases are those in which the patient has her first cesarean operation. For many years, it was thought that once a woman had had a C-section, she could no longer deliver vaginally without danger of uterine rupture. According to this reasoning, once a woman had had one C-section, subsequent deliveries would automatically be done surgically.

In many areas of the country, obstetricians still refuse to do vaginal deliveries on patients who have previously had an abdominal delivery. Though that philosophy is a minority viewpoint, it probably is not fair at this time to evaluate a doctor's section rate by including the repeat cases. Until more of a consensus is achieved, many doctors are afraid that if complications occur during vaginal delivery, they may be subject to claims for malpractice. Many of these women can and should be delivered vaginally; and in the not too distant future, this will be the accepted practice. The obstetrical literature is now filled with information expressing that opinion. The primary C-section rate is much more within control of the doctor.

What is reasonable?

No one has yet determined what the proper rate of primary C-sections should be. However, various studies and reports indicate that:

1. *Some breech babies* should be delivered by C-section. Factors to be considered are the size of the baby, the position of the baby's legs, the size of the mother's pelvis, the progress of the labor, and the baby's well being as determined by monitoring during labor. Since some breech babies can be delivered vaginally, doctors who deliver all by C-section are doing too many.

2. Some women who have had *previous C-sections* will need to have them again. Factors to be considered are the reasons for the first operation as well as current conditions. Since some previously sectioned women can deliver vaginally, doctors sectioning all of them are doing too many.

3. Some women undergoing a *long, slow labor* will need to have a C-section. Factors to be considered should be the size of the pelvic opening, the size and position of the baby, and the quality of the contractions in labor. With patience and proper treatment such as sedation, fluids, rest, ambulation, and the use of medication to improve labor, many women in prolonged labor can be delivered vaginally. Doctors doing cesareans in all of these cases are doing too many.

4. *Fetal distress* is a proper indication for C-section. However, doctors who perform C-sections at the slightest suspicion of fetal distress (even though procedures are available to provide greater information that may demonstrate that true distress may not be present) are doing too many.

5. Some doctors do C-sections for their own convenience, and a few even do them for financial gain.

An interesting study has been done in Australia on two groups of women, one of which had many more specialists caring for them than the other. The C-section rate in the specialist group was 12 to 14 percent, considerably higher than that of the group without specialists. The researchers found that the newborn survival rate for both groups was approximately the same. The higher C-section rate among those treated by the specialists had not resulted in any improvement in newborn survival.

Although the technique of C-section has improved greatly, it is important to remember that complications still occur. A 1978 editorial in the *Canadian Medical Association Journal* noted that maternal deaths from C-sections occurred 26 times as often as those from vaginal delivery. Even when the women who had serious pre-existing disease were not counted, the mortality rate for C-sections was still 10 times as great as that for vaginal deliveries. The authors of the editorial concluded that doctors should not take the "easy way out of a difficult delivery" without considering the subsequent risks. Increased risk to the mother could be justified only if infant survival rates were significantly improved by cesarean delivery.

In 1980, a more comprehensive study by the National Institutes of Health reported a corrected maternal mortality rate 2 to 4 times higher in C-sections than in vaginal deliveries.

Why the C-section rate is rising

From 1965 to 1971, the rate of C-sections rose only from 4.6 to 5.5 percent of deliveries. Since that time, however, the increase has been 10 to 20 percent per year, so that by

1981, the nationwide rate had reached 19.3 percent. A number of researchers have attempted to identify the causes for this rising rate. The Canadian Medical Association editorial analyzed this issue well when it cited the following factors:

1. Increased use of continuous fetal monitoring—a method of identifying complications to the unborn fetus during labor.

2. An increase in the proportion of women having their first baby. These patients have the highest rate of C-section.

3. The increasing belief that delivery by C-section is safer than certain types of vaginal breech delivery.

4. More aggressive use of C-section in the treatment of toxemia of pregnancy—a condition which threatens the welfare and survival of both mother and baby.

5. With the improved survival rates of very small babies (those delivered as early as the 28th week of pregnancy), there is an increasing indication for these to be delivered by C-section because the trauma of labor and delivery may be too great for very small premature babies.

6. A changing attitude towards labor—and whether it presents additional risks. For example, a course of labor which lasts longer than average may make the physician inclined to operate.

7. A massive increase in malpractice suits has made many physicians feel extremely insecure. If an injury is present at birth, parents may sue the physician on the theory that the problem would not have occurred had a C-section been done. This situation makes some doctors extra-quick to operate—for what they believe are *legal* rather than medical reasons! Unfortunately, this problem cannot be solved by doctors alone. It will continue—and may even get worse—unless state lawmakers find ways to protect conscientious doctors from *unfair* malpractice suits.

8. An increasing number of repeat C-sections, which is the natural outcome of an increasing number of primary sections for the indications already mentioned.

In 1980, three doctors published a report of definite improvement in fetal and maternal death rates as the rate of C-sections rose. But they still felt that the rate might be lowered somewhat if physicians did two things. Better management of labor might correct some of the problems associated with poor progress in labor (dystocia); and the old cardinal rule, "Once a section, always a section," should be reevaluated.

The latest information appears to demonstrate that the 5 percent C-section rates of 20 years ago are too low, and that obstetrical care has improved considerably as the section rate has risen. Whether the correct overall rate should be 10, 15 or 20 percent is not yet medically settled. But cases of abuse can still be identified.

The dark side of the increase

I believe that most practicing obstetricians are doing a fine job of deciding when C-sections are necessary. However, when that decision is made improperly, what factors are involved? The truth is a painful pill, since the reasons are atrocious:

1. Cesarean section is a relatively simple operation. Performing it early in labor relieves the involved physician from having to wait for spontaneous labor to be completed.

2. A delivery may be somewhat more difficult than average, but not to the point of danger to the baby. The physician may be so insecure in his ability to perform that procedure that he avoids it by doing a C-section.

3. The fee for a C-section is higher than that for a vaginal delivery. Logically that may make little sense, since the time and ability necessary for vaginal delivery may be considerably greater.

Picture this not-very-rare scenario: The patient is admitted at 7:00 a.m. The doctor stimulates her labor while at the same time scheduling her for a C-section at 5:30 p.m. If the patient is lucky and has all the various factors (size of pelvis, size of baby, efficiency of labor) aligned just perfectly, she will deliver before the scheduled time for the operation. If, however, she is among the group who commonly take much longer than that to complete their labor, she most likely will be subjected to a C-section that evening—for the doctor's convenience!

Except for previously scheduled C-sections, which are

usually done in the early morning, by far the greatest number are done immediately after office hours. There is no doubt in my mind that appropriate watchful waiting would allow many of these women to deliver vaginally. Deliveries would then occur, however, at much less convenient times for the doctor.

Fetal monitoring

One of the factors related to the rising C-section rate has been the advent of continuous fetal monitoring. This involves the use of electrical devices to keep track of the frequency and duration of the uterine contractions and the heart rate of the fetus. Additional equipment can be used to measure the strength of the contractions, but this is not widely done. It is also possible to evaluate the condition of the baby by measuring the acidity (pH) of the baby's blood. This is accomplished by testing a blood specimen from the baby's scalp obtained via the mother's vagina during labor.

These methods now enable doctors to determine with ease, and generally quite early in labor, when a baby is becoming distressed. It is then possible to decide whether continuing the labor will be dangerous to the unborn child and whether a C-section done immediately might make the difference between life and death.

When fetal monitoring equipment was introduced, it was generally used only on certain categories of high-risk patients. But as time passed, doctors came to believe that even mothers and babies with no obvious risk factors might undergo a sudden change during labor which could cause the death of the child. As a result, more and more patients were placed on fetal monitors. Today almost all patients are monitored.

Some authorities believe that routine use of monitoring is the main factor in the increased incidence of C-sections. If only numbers are considered, this claim appears to be accurate. But a closer look indicates that the equipment is not to blame.

During labor, changes occur repeatedly on the monitors. Many are not serious and in fact may be reversed by simple techniques. It has been demonstrated clearly that having a patient turn from a position flat on her back to either left or right side can usually cause abnormal fetal heart rates to disappear. Administering oxygen may also help the heartbeat to return to a normal rate. But some obstetricians use the slightest change on the monitor as an excuse for performing a C-section.

For other doctors the effect has been quite the reverse. In the past, it was automatically assumed that a long labor indicated increased risk to the baby. Before the advent of continuous monitoring, doctors often felt pressured in these cases to go directly to a C-section. Today, although a long labor might portend problems in some cases, it is certainly not dangerous for all. Many women will deliver vaginally quite easily if their doctors have the patience to wait for the necessary progress. For these doctors, monitoring has created the opportunity to wait longer with confidence that the baby is not in danger. Thus it is clear that although fetal monitoring can change C-section rates, the direction of the change is more a reflection of the doctor than of the equipment.

Survey of a major hospital

In the hospital which I evaluated, during a 1-year period the primary C-section rate was 13.8 percent and the rate for repeat C-section was 6.5 percent of total deliveries. Proper evaluation of previously sectioned women would have considerable impact on the overall C-section rate. But for now we shall deal only with the rate of primary C-sections.

Since the decision to do an abdominal delivery most often involves women having their first child, one might expect doctors who were new in their practice to have high C-section rates. They are more likely than established obstetricians to have a higher percentage of women in their first pregnancy. However, in this evaluation, the C-section rates for the new physicians in the community were generally the lower percentage figures. Thus, the overall rate apparently was not affected by the fact that some physicians attended more women having their first deliveries. During the 1-year period, 2,514 deliveries were performed by the 20 obstetricians I studied. Table 5:1 summarizes my findings:

Table 5:1. Primary cesarean rates for different doctors in 1981

Doctor	Patients in labor	Number of cesareans	Percentage cesareans
A	217	15	6.9
B	113	8	7.1
C	114	9	7.9
D	208	20	9.6
E	112	12	10.7
F	74	8	10.8
G	149	17	11.4
H	95	11	11.6
I	50	6	12.0
J	410	53	12.9
K	45	6	13.3
L	67	9	13.4
M	95	13	13.7
N	99	14	14.1
O	106	16	15.1
P	74	13	17.6
Q	189	40	21.2
R	106	23	21.7
S	145	36	24.8
T	46	17	37.0
TOTAL	2,514	346	13.8

It could be argued that some doctors on this list may have done too few C-sections and that their patients might have had better care had their rate been slightly higher. But I believe those doctors having the lower section rates were practicing a high quality of medical care. I have observed them carefully attending to their patients and performing C-sections only when there were clear and logical reasons to do so.

Of the 20 physicians studied, 4 had a primary C-section rate under 10 percent, while 11 others had rates between 10 and 15 percent. Certainly all of those numbers come reasonably close to each other and demonstrate a rather clear pattern of what an acceptable primary C-section rate should be in today's medical environment. We are left then with Drs. P through T, who delivered 21 percent of the babies at the hospital.

The lowest primary section rate for that group was 17.5 percent. One might be hard-pressed to make a definitive statement that the number was sufficiently beyond the great majority to be classified outright excessive. There is little doubt, however, about the others.

Doctors Q, R and S had rates of 21.3, 21.7, and 24.8 percent. That means they were performing primary C-sections on one out of every four or five women in labor. If we examine the same information for those doctors who were doing the other 81 percent of the deliveries at that institution, their primary rate was 11.3 percent. They operated on one out of nine women in labor.

Worst of all, Doctor T, unpoliced, unrestricted, yet well known among his colleagues for his inadequate care, had a primary C-section rate of 37 percent. More than one out of every three of Dr. T's patients in labor ends up on the operating room table, subjected to major surgery, anesthesia, prolonged hospitalization, loss of time, and increased expense! Doctors jest among themselves about his inept medical performance, but the "old-boy" community takes no action to stop it. So he continues to practice, and his patients—blissfully unaware of the risks to which they are exposed—think he is wonderful.

Physicians in positions of authority will state that nothing can be done to curb the abuses. I certainly disagree! I believe that it is the obligation of *doctors* to take action. Hospital staffs can practice stringent peer review and take action to prevent obvious patterns of abuse from continuing. But the sad fact is that effective policing action is rarely taken by doctors against doctors, lawyers against lawyers, police against police, or for that matter, within any other professional group.

If one takes as an average what the other hospital physicians established as a fairly normal primary C-section rate (a number which would appear to be quite proper in relation to the national average), one would find that approximately 70 women could be estimated as having had unnecessary C-sections in the hands of those five doctors.

That number is approximately 20 percent of all the abdominal deliveries performed there. That computation assumes, probably overgenerously, that in all the remaining deliveries done by the other ¾ths of the physicians at the hospital, there was not a single case of an unnecessary C-section. My research found that the doctors with the highest C-section rates are the ones who overutilize other types of gynecological surgery.

It can be difficult or even impossible to determine whether C-section was necessary by looking back on individual cases. However, doctors who are doing too high a percentage *overall* can be detected by conscientious peer review and then watched closely to *prevent* further abuses.

When I showed my data to a number of ethical physicians at the hospital in which the data were collected, their responses were shock and disbelief. Even they did not realize how bad the situation had become. But the situation had evolved only because of their subconscious decision *not to be involved*. They themselves practiced obstetrics properly (as they knew they must). Whatever was going on around them was "not their problem." Yet they knew what the C-section rate for the hospital had become, and that their own rates were far below that. Simple mathematics made it certain that someone had to be raising the average!

In 1983, I repeated my study and found that the situation has been getting worse. The primary C-section rate had risen from 13.8 percent to 19.7 percent—and the overall section rate was over 28 percent!

Two of the original 20 physicians had stopped practicing obstetrics and 15 new obstetricians had joined the staff. Of the five highest listed in the chart, Dr. S had reduced his primary C-section rate to just below 20 percent. Drs. P, Q, R and T were now 24.2, 33.3, 21.3 and 34.6 percent, respectively. One other physician whose case load had been small had soared to a primary C-section rate of 42.2 percent! Of the newcomers, most were in a reasonable range, but four had primary C-section rates over 25 percent. The doctors with primary rates over 24.2 percent performed 41 percent of the C-sections although they did only 29 percent of the deliveries. Their average primary C-section rate was 28 percent, in contrast to the rest of the staff who averaged 16.4 percent.

Unhappily, these figures are probably typical. The hospitals I have observed personally are high-quality institutions, fully accredited and considered by physicians and patients in their communities to be among the best in their respective areas. I believe that the numbers above—and worse—can be reproduced in many hospitals throughout the country.

Second opinion?

Beyond the numbers is a sham which often accompanies them. Many hospitals require that a second doctor be called as a consultant in the decision to perform a primary cesarean section. Does this negate the validity of the above data, or indicate that all of the consulting individuals were involved in the abuse? Neither is actually the case.

The truth is that the consultation is meaningless and valueless. No one actually calls another doctor in *for consultation*. The second doctor is asked to sign a form stating that he concurs with the decision to operate. He does no examination, and in fact, customarily does not even see the patient until he enters the operating suite to assist. In his own mind, the second doctor comes only to help in the surgical procedure and signs the form only to fulfill the hospital requirements. No one actually asks that doctor to make any *judgment*. Surgical procedures are done routinely without second opinions. What makes this process distasteful is the phony appearance that a second opinion has been sought and given.

At a recent seminar, Dr. John T. Queenan, Chairman of the Department of Obstetrics and Gynecology at Georgetown University School of Medicine, put forth a strategy for reducing the C-section rate:

1. A hospital policy of consultation for failure of labor to progress or for fetal distress. (These would be *true* second opinions.)

2. Fetal scalp blood sampling to accurately assess whether the fetus is in distress.

3. Departmental review of all first-time cesarean sections.

4. Monitoring of staff patterns with respect to the frequency of cesareans. (This would identify specific offenders.)

It would not be surprising to see such actions have a worthwhile effect. An audit of C-sections in Scotland reported in 1982 demonstrated the sentinel effect clearly. Once doctors knew a study was being done, the rate—which had increased steadily for the previous 10 years—decreased.

This, then, is the status of cesarean section. The patient in the labor room is completely at the mercy of her doctor. Abusive doctors can be controlled only by conscientious supervision by other doctors.

6

OTHER QUESTIONABLE OPERATIONS

This chapter discusses a variety of diseases of the ovaries and Fallopian tubes which can lead to surgery. In each of these conditions, the patient may be told by the doctor that surgery is needed to save her life or to determine whether a life-threatening condition is present. In some of these cases, surgery is clearly justified. In others it may be a close question, but often surgery can be avoided through conservative management or the use of appropriate diagnostic tests.

The ovaries, located on each side of the lower abdomen near the uterus, are almond-shaped and usually measure about 1 by 1½ inches. They release eggs (ovulate), usually on a cyclic basis, about once a month. They also function as part of the reproductive hormonal system and secrete the female hormones, estrogen and progesterone. The Fallopian tubes (often simply referred to as the "tubes") are tubular structures approximately 3 to 5 inches long and ¼- to ½-inch in diameter through which the eggs can travel from ovaries to uterus.

During the normal menstrual cycle, women develop a structure on the ovary subsequent to ovulation. That structure, known as a corpus luteum, frequently develops into a cyst (a fluid-filled sac). The cyst may appear as anything from a slight enlargement of the ovary to one of considerable size. Most corpus luteum cysts cause no significant problems. Even large ones usually recede by themselves without treatment. If they rupture and bleed, except in the rarest of cases, that bleeding will be self-limiting with no need for surgery.

Ovaries can develop a wide variety of enlargements, ranging from large, solid cancers to many different types of benign or malignant cysts. The most common type of ovarian enlargement, however, is the corpus luteum cyst.

Diagnostic procedures

Many patients who seek medical attention for pelvic pain are discovered by the doctor to have an ovarian cyst. It is common practice for these patients to be told that their pain is caused by the presence of that cyst and that they must undergo exploratory abdominal surgery (laparotomy). Sometimes they are told that surgery is necessary to be sure that no cancer is present. This advice may be correct. However, in many cases, a thorough diagnostic evaluation would make it clear that neither cancer nor any other condition is present which requires surgery.

Most of these women who are incorrectly advised to have surgery are young. This is because young women often develop harmless corpus luteum cysts due to hormonal imbalance. To determine the appropriate course of action, doctors can use the following diagnostic procedures.

Bimanual examination is a technique of pelvic examination in which the doctor inserts one finger into the woman's vagina or rectum and presses on the woman's abdomen with the fingers of the other hand. Each ovary can actually be located and held between the hands, enabling the doctor to determine whether it is tender, enlarged, or abnormally hard.

Although ovarian cancer is not rare, the great majority of ovarian enlargements are noncancerous. Sometimes it is difficult to tell whether a mass is benign or malignant from a single examination. Findings which would tend to make a doctor want to operate after a single examination include:

1) a mass over 2½ inches in diameter
2) a solid mass (verified by ultrasound examination)
3) increasing enlargement of the abdomen
4) accumulation of blood or other fluid inside the abdomen
5) ovarian enlargement in a postmenopausal woman.

On the other hand, a mass that is smaller or feels cystic, especially one in a premenopausal woman under the age of 35, can be followed with re-examination in 4 to 6 weeks to determine whether it has enlarged. In the majority of cases, the mass will have disappeared. Even if it remains and the examiner is uncertain about its consistency, exploratory abdominal surgery should not be the first step. An ultrasound study or laparoscopy (described below) ought to shed light on the severity of the problem.

Culdocentesis is a technique in which a needle is inserted through the back of the vagina into the abdominal cavity to discern how much, if any, free blood is present in the abdomen. This procedure produces only minimal to moderate amount of pain and can almost always be done with local anesthesia or no anesthesia.

Laparoscopy is a procedure in which the doctor looks into the abdominal cavity through an instrument and can make a judgment without having the patient undergo major surgery. This technique can be done in a short-stay surgical unit and does not usually require an overnight stay in the hospital.

Sonography (often referred to as "ultrasound") is a technique which uses sound waves to generate a picture of the structures in the abdomen. It can demonstrate the density of the structures and whether their size is normal or increased.

Pregnancy testing is important because it helps the doctor decide whether the problem is a complication of pregnancy (such as an ectopic pregnancy) or another type of condition such as an ovarian cyst. The test can be done on a specimen of blood or urine.

An important study

Ruptured or unruptured corpus luteum cysts often occur in the early stages of pregnancy. These usually have no serious consequences, but may be confused with ectopic pregnancy (discussed below). In both conditions, the patient may have pain, a palpable mass in the area of the tube and ovary, and a positive pregnancy test. In these cases, culdocentesis and if necessary, laparoscopy, can clarify the diagnosis when it is not obvious from physical examination.

In the November, 1979 issue of the *American Journal of Obstetrics and Gynecology*, Dr. Lester T. Hibbard of the Department of OB/Gyn, University of Southern California, reported on 200 women who were found at surgery to have a corpus luteum cyst. Ninety-two percent were between the ages of 16 and 30.

Almost all of these patients had sought treatment because of pain, and the majority of them had missed a menstrual period. In some of the cases, the examining doctor felt something abnormal on pelvic examination, either an abnormal mass or an area of fullness which suggested that internal bleeding had taken place. Unruptured corpus luteum cysts almost never require abdominal surgery (laparotomy). However, ruptured corpus luteum cysts with *uncontrollable* bleeding do require surgery, although most ruptured cysts are not accompanied by such severe bleeding and can be managed by laparoscopy and watchful waiting.

Dr. Hibbard's analysis was quite complicated and technical, but two statistics are especially significant. First, 37 of the 200 patients—who showed little or no bleeding on culdocentesis—needed no surgery at all! Second, of 150 women with negative pregnancy tests and records complete enough to analyze, 114 did not need laparotomy but could have been diagnosed with laparoscopy alone after the diagnosis was made with pregnancy testing and culdocentesis.

I, too, have observed cases of other doctors in which surgery could have been avoided with adequate diagnostic testing or a longer period of observation.

It would be unreasonable to expect doctors to be 100 percent accurate in diagnosing possible corpus luteum cysts. However, appropriate evaluation using the above-described techniques allows the ethical physician to explain to the patient that the most beneficial form of treatment in many cases is "watchful waiting." Most women with symptomatic corpus luteum cysts will recover spontaneously if given the time. Physicians who perform these operations excessively may account for their actions by saying that they are afraid of missing a cancer or ruptured ectopic pregnancy. We know, however, that the risk of malignancy is low in young women.

Over the years, many parents have asked my advice when their daughter who is away at school has been told she has an ovarian cyst that requires surgery. Since few ovarian cysts in young women actually require surgery, I advise getting a second opinion. In the cases brought to me for that opinion, I have rarely found a reason to operate. *Young women who are seen for the first time by a gynecologist who tells them to have surgery for an ovarian cyst should be very wary and seek a second opinion!*

The cost of unnecessary ovarian surgery can be quite high. Dr. Hibbard found that the average length of hospital stay for laparoscopy was 1.2 days and the average for laparotomy was 4.3 days. In addition to the daily room rate, patients must pay for the operating room and anesthesia plus a surgical fee of $500 to $1,000 for laparoscopy or twice that for laparotomy. I believe that money is a definite factor in the decision of some doctors to operate unnecessarily in these cases.

Ectopic pregnancy

An ectopic pregnancy is a gestation found outside of its normal location within the uterus. The condition occurs as a result of the inability of an egg, fertilized in the Fallopian tube, to make its way down the tube into the uterine cavity where it is supposed to implant itself in the uterine lining. The inability is usually caused by scarring in the tube from a previous infection, or an anatomical defect in the tube which traps the egg and does not allow it to pass. Most ectopic pregnancies are located in one of the Fallopian tubes and are not capable of going to full term. Generally they rupture out of the thin-walled tube and into the abdominal cavity if not diagnosed early enough.

If ectopic pregnancy is found, surgery is always necessary. The diagnosis can be difficult to make before the rupture occurs and frequently will not be made until that point. If the rupture is significant, the diagnosis is usually obvious and surgery should be instituted immediately to control the internal bleeding.

Prior to rupture, the diagnosis can be made if there is reason to suspect that something unusual is brewing. In such cases, many of the same tests discussed in the section on ovarian cysts may be utilized.

In its classic form, a ruptured ectopic pregnancy manifests symptoms which are clearly recognizable: severe pain in the abdomen, at times referred to the shoulders, an acutely tender abdomen, weakness and fainting due to blood loss, in a woman who has missed a period or has irregular menstrual cycles. These cases are emergencies and must have surgery quickly. The question of unnecessary surgery does not apply here. Symptoms reaching that severity indicate that a large amount of bleeding has taken place within the abdomen. Even if the diagnosis is inaccurate, and the large amount of bleeding is from a rare case of ruptured corpus luteum cyst, it will still be necessary to operate to control the bleeding from that source.

A difficult situation occurs with the diagnosis of a possible unruptured ectopic pregnancy. Here the patient may have a positive or even a negative pregnancy test, some minimal to moderate pain and tenderness, and missing or irregular menses.

Unfortunately, many of these patients diagnosed as having an "ectopic pregnancy" turn out to have no such condition when the abdomen is opened. Often there is present an intrauterine pregnancy with a small cyst in the ovary. There may also be a persistent corpus luteum which, by disturbing the hormonal balance, has delayed the next menstrual cycle and confused the clinical picture. Though that delay will not be accompanied by a positive pregnancy test, the existence of the menstrual irregularity combined with some discomfort and the presence of a palpable mass can lead a physician who is unwilling to diligently observe and monitor the patient to perform unnecessary major surgery. There is no danger, however, with either the small cyst during pregnancy or the persistent corpus luteum, and absolutely no need for surgery.

The patient and her family, in their naiveté, are pleased and relieved when the doctor comes out after the operation to tell them how lucky they were that there was no ectopic pregnancy. He reveals that there was an ovarian cyst which he gallantly removed to "save the day." No one ever thinks to discuss whether or not he should have operated at all.

A problem also arises with hospital peer review: the fact that the "necessity" is based only on a preoperative diagnosis of ectopic gestation, *even if that diagnosis is not correct.* Never does the concept of proper preoperative evaluation of the condition come into play. Never does anyone ever judge whether the physician has adequate reason to be going ahead with the surgical procedure. No one is even concerned about whether some physicians make that *mis*diagnosis repeatedly. Once the diagnosis of "possible ectopic pregnancy" appears on the chart it is automatically accepted for whatever treatment is utilized.

Failure of peer review

Not every gynecologist rushes in to operate on all of these patients, but Dr. Hibbard's research should provide some insight. Obviously, the number who do cannot be insignificant. If there are only a small percentage of doctors doing these cases, why aren't they identified and controlled by their peers? The answer remains the same. The medical profession will not adequately police itself.

These cases may be handled by using the types of evaluation described by Dr. Hibbard: observation, blood tests, pregnancy tests, culdocentesis, and finally laparoscopy if the diagnosis is still not clear. As stated previously, the obvious ruptured ectopics need not be pre-evaluated by laparoscopy or second opinion.

Even the most honest and ethical gynecologist will at times operate and find no significant problem. Some cases are extremely difficult and confusing and not resolvable by any means we possess. It is unrealistic to believe that physicians could avoid every case that might have been handled nonsurgically. However, as noted in Chapter 9, my study of cases diagnosed preoperatively as "ectopic pregnancy" at a Texas hospital during 1981 uncovered a serious problem. Some doctors who failed to do sufficient diagnostic testing were accurate only 25 percent of the time or less. Obviously, some of these cases where no ectopic pregnancy was present could have been handled without "the knife." In many of them, the above-mentioned tests were not even utilized. And a second opinion from a qualified gynecologist might also have averted some of the operations.

Opponents of this position might state that delay will result in true unruptured ectopic pregnancies rupturing before surgery. That possibility exists. However, most ectopic pregnancies are not diagnosed until they have ruptured to some extent. The delay involved in doing proper testing is unlikely to cause the condition to progress to rupture. It is usually the case in which no one suspects any abnormality that ultimately results in rupture.

7

EXCESSIVE TESTING

S o far this book has been focused on the overuse of surgical procedures within obstetrics and gynecology.
This emphasis is proper because these procedures
threaten the health of the women exposed to them. Now
let's look at other abuses whose impact is primarily economic: the excessive use of Pap smears, colposcopy, ultrasound, and a variety of other diagnostic procedures. All
of these tests are *extremely* valuable when used
appropriately—but, as with many medical advances,
excesses and abuses can occur as a result of ignorance,
overzealousness or greed.

The Pap Smear

During the past two years, a severe conflict has broken
out within medical ranks. The American Cancer Society
and The American College of Obstetrics and Gynecology,
which previously had agreed about the frequency of Pap
smears, are now at odds on that issue. This conflict did
not arise out of a sudden, remarkable discovery. A major
abuse is at its heart.

The Pap smear is named after its developer, pathologist
Dr. George Papanicolaou, who announced in 1928 that he

had developed a technique for identifying certain characteristics of cells from a vaginal smear. Cells shed from the lining of the cervix and vagina are examined under a microscope after a chemical fixative has been applied to maintain them in a relatively permanent condition. The appearance of the cells can indicate when cancer is present or may be developing. The test is only a screening procedure. When the cells look suspicious, more definitive testing must be done to determine the exact nature of the problem.

Development of the Pap smear has revolutionized the management of the cervix. Prior to the test's use, cancer of the cervix was more common and killed more people than cancer of the uterus. Today, because of this marvelous tool, cancer of the cervix is being detected *before* it develops, and cancer of the uterus is the more common.

Research involving the Pap smear has proven that cervical cancer is a slow-growing process in which cervical cells undergo pre-malignant changes long before the actual life-threatening malignant state develops. As a result of this insight, women were encouraged to have an annual Pap smear which could reveal an approaching malignancy at a preventable stage. (In fact, if every woman took adequate measures, cervical cancer would almost cease to exist.) Women at almost every level of our society became aware of this advance, and to a great extent took advantage of that opportunity to protect themselves. Then the trouble began: some doctors used the procedure to draw patients to their offices more often than is medically necessary. This was easy to do because their patients thought that greater frequency meant greater safety from cervical cancer.

During the 23 years that I have been doing Pap smears, I have not seen a single patient whose Pap smear revealed actual cancer of the cervix who had had a normal Pap smear the year before. In every cancer case, the patient had either gone for many years without a Pap smear or had had an abnormal smear previously. There have been rare reports of patients with a normal Pap smear who were found to have cervical cancer within one year. In such situations the initial smear may have been in error or some extraordinary change may have occurred.

Regardless of the cause, that situation is so rare that no logical person would suggest that we do routine Pap smears more frequently than once a year. The cost in relation to the risk factor would be astronomical. It would be no more logical than suggesting that all people should have the brake linings of their car checked every month to detect a change before a critical level is reached. To evaluate any type of preventive measure, both cost and effectiveness must be taken into consideration.

It doesn't take a very astute or mathematical mind to realize that doctors who check their patients every six months will gross twice as much money from checkups as doctors who see their patients once a year.

In recent years, the number of gynecologists serving middle and upper economic metropolitan areas has been increasing so that there are fewer patients per doctor. To maintain their income, some physicians advise *normal* women to be examined twice a year instead of annually. Some doctors are less blatant than others and advise this checkup schedule for only certain patients: those taking birth control pills or those over the age of 40. These groups, of course, comprise a major portion of their patients.

It was this type of abuse that ultimately led to the study by the American Cancer Society (ACS) to determine how frequently Pap smears should be performed. It now recommends an annual Pap smear for women beyond the age of 40. Women between 20 and 40 and those sexually active under the age of 20 are advised to have Pap smears at least once every three years after they have had two negative Pap smears one year apart. Note that the ACS wording is flexible. It does not state that three years should be the definitive interval in these patients, but only that three years should be the maximum interval. In cases where there is no abnormal history, the ACS advocates that Pap smears should not be performed more often than once a year. More frequent smears may be necessary when there is an abnormal or questionable Pap report.

The resistance to this position has been quite strong. The American College of Obstetrics and Gynecology still recommends that *routine* Pap smears be obtained annually on women between the ages of 20 and 40. Some doctors even advise having them every six months. Only patients can control this problem.

As women enter their thirties, it may be prudent to have their breast and pelvic examinations annually. However, this does not mean that a Pap smear is necessary every time as part of the physical checkup.

Actually, the entire concept of preventive checkups is being re-evaluated by ethical physicians. Routine chest x-ray examinations for screening purposes have generally been abandoned except for certain high-risk individuals. Recently the AMA suggested that the interval for complete physical exams should be every five years in apparently healthy young adults. Rational guidelines for the frequency of mammography, sigmoidoscopy, electrocardiograms and various other tests and procedures are being developed. How well the medical community will accept these suggestions remains to be seen. Prudent consumers should become familiar with these guidelines and the reasons behind them.

Some gynecologists claim that it is urgent to examine women on birth control pills every six months to identify the development of high blood pressure which can occur in some cases. If hypertension were found, the pill would be stopped—as it should be. However, a doctor who is really concerned about this problem can simply have his patients return every six months for a blood pressure check by his nurse. Extra pelvic examinations and Pap smears are unnecessary.

To make matters worse, victims of unnecessary Pap smears may be led to believe they are receiving the very best of care in the form of "close medical supervision"! Most gynecologists do *not* ask their patients to return more often than once a year. However, the ethical majority is a *silent* majority whose failure to speak out permits unhindered abuse by the unethical minority.

Medical apathy

At a meeting whose subject matter should have attracted the most sophisticated physicians, I attended a roundtable luncheon with nine other gynecologists who were strangers to me. Somehow the conversation got around to the ethics of medical practice. Only one other physician supported my view that it was unethical to bring disease-free patients back to the office on a 6-month basis. Two doctors who were partners had the honesty and gall to say that if they didn't practice that way, their office hours would not be sufficiently full and they "wouldn't make enough money." I believe that this sentiment—though seldom discussed publicly—is not rare.

I was even more disturbed by a situation which existed while I was co-director of an Ob/Gyn department in a major metropolitan hospital. A county Ob-Gyn society had been created to provide education and guidance to its physician members. I contacted the president and encouraged him to take an official stand to the effect that acceptable practice does not include the encouraging of excessive visits to the gynecologist. Except where specific conditions exist which would necessitate more frequent observation, an annual checkup and Pap smear would be more than sufficient. To my dismay, he refused to speak out to the membership.

Diethylstilbestrol (DES)

The diagnosis and treatment of cancer of the vagina in young women whose mothers received DES during their pregnancy is confused by emotional overtones. Diethylstilbestrol is a synthetic hormone which has little usefulness today.

Over 30 years ago, it was thought that pregnant women who were threatening to miscarry, as demonstrated by bleeding during the first three months of pregnancy, might avoid that outcome by using DES. Its use at that time was based on several published studies which suggested that DES might help to prevent and treat threatened abortions and a number of other complications of pregnancy. This material was then supported by anecdotal reports of its value. Although one well-designed study in 1953 suggested that miscarriages would not be prevented by the administration of DES, doctors felt they had much to gain and little to lose by trying it. Its use continued until 1970 when, for the first time, two pathologists began reporting an association between vaginal cancer and maternal exposure to DES.

Looking back at this situation, it is clear that the use of DES in these mothers was an extremely unfortunate error. Although better research, done earlier, would have revealed the lack of value in its use, the disastrous long-range effect could not have been predicted.

Millions of women took DES as advised by their physicians. It is extremely important to understand that since this treatment was generally accepted by the medical community, patients had very little option other than to accept it. *It is unfair to place any blame for this outcome on the patient.* It would be comparable to expecting a patient suffering with a critical case of pneumonia to reject antibiotic therapy on the fantastically unlikely premise that 20 years from now it would result in a cancer.

Why do I bring up the issue of "fault"? Actually, that is a basic point in understanding what is happening now, 20 or more years after the fact. A psychological environment has been created in which women who received this medication have been made to feel responsible for the outcome. They have not only been anxiously attempting to find out whether they received DES (a worthwhile endeavor); many of them have also been requesting overtreatment for their daughters because of encouragement they are receiving from some physicians and organizations.

It is not too difficult to induce people to accept a treatment if they believe that avoiding the treatment will endanger their health. In the same way, it is easy to encourage testing if a mother feels guilty for possibly jeopardizing her child's health and life. Under these circumstances, what parent is likely to refuse anything that might appear to counteract such a problem?

Recent data indicate that the frequency of vaginal malignancy in "DES daughters" is in the range of 1 in 4,000. That incidence is far less than the risk of cancer of the cervix faced by *every* woman. As stated previously, women who have normal vaginal examinations and Pap smears need those procedures repeated no more often than once a year.

Colposcopy is a procedure in which the cervix and vagina are examined with a special microscope to look for cancer. There is no valid reason to use colposcopy to look for cancer unless a woman's Pap smear is abnormal. Despite the extremely low risk which daughters of DES recipients face, some doctors advise them—in the absence of abnormal findings—to have Pap smears every six months, colposcopy (at times repeated at subsequent visits), and even vaginal biopsies with no specific indication. No research findings justify such advice.

A 1982 survey of gynecologists in a large Texas community found that most advise managing DES daughters in the same way as non-DES-exposed patients—which is the accepted scientific viewpoint. But more than 25 percent of the surveyed physicians indicated that they order excessive treatment either in the form of visits every 6 months or an immediate colposcopy even when the Pap smear and examination are normal.

Researchers have found that DES-exposed women have a higher incidence of pelvic anatomical abnormalities that do non-exposed women. During the past five years, several studies have demonstrated that DES daughters have a higher than average incidence of anatomical deformities of the uterus as well as a higher risk of fetal loss through miscarriage, premature labor or ectopic pregnancy (pregnancy outside of the uterus). These findings have stimulated some gynecologists to subject DES daughters to hysterosalpingography, a special x-ray study. In this test, a special dye visible on x-ray films is inserted into the cervical canal, passes upward to the uterus and Fallopian tubes, and highlights anatomical problems which might interfere with pregnancy.

This approach is irrational! Recent studies by Dr. Ann Barnes of Harvard Medical School have revealed no significant difference in fertility between DES daughters and non-exposed women. Even if DES daughters did have more difficulty, it is absurd to subject them to such testing unless they experience difficulty in becoming pregnant.

Though hysterosalpingography is fairly safe, a few women experience allergic reactions to the dye—and unnecessary radiation should always be avoided.

Abuse of sophisticated equipment

A potential problem exists for several types of expensive medical equipment that physicians may use in their offices. Two prime examples are the colposcope and the ultrasound machine. Both of these devices are exceedingly valuable when used appropriately and have been responsible for remarkable improvements in patient care. The questions at hand, however, are which patients should have such testing—and who should do it?

There is no question whatsoever that gynecologists who concentrate their practice in the area of malignancy must have a colposcope. They should develop great expertise in its use or they will not perform their job adequately. Similarly, obstetricians who deal mainly in high-risk pregnancies might need their own ultrasound equipment. But most obstetricians and gynecologists do not direct their practices primarily to either of those fields.

The equipment salesman who comes to the office on a regular basis attempting to sell his wares plays a role in this problem. The salesman will provide the doctor with complete information about how the equipment works and the good it can provide. In almost every pitch, however, he will attempt to clinch the sale on an economic basis. He expects the doctor to say "$3,000 (or $5,000, $10,000 or $20,000) is a lot of money for me to spend for that." The salesman will then respond with how much of a moneymaker the instrument will be: "Don't you know that insurance companies will pay $75 (or $90, $100, or $150) every time the procedure is done. Only 50, 100, or what you could do in a year, and the equipment will be paid for. The rest will be profit."

In a recent advertisement for an obstetrical monitoring device for the office, well over half the information provided dealt with the financial advantages of its purchase. How often do you think equipment companies or their salespeople concern themselves with whether potential customers actually *need* the equipment?

Once an expensive piece of equipment has been bought, financial considerations will entice the doctor to use it. In the case of the colposcope, some physicians recommend colposcopy on an annual basis for all patients beyond a certain age. Some will perform it even with a negative Pap smear. These practices are improper.

In my own practice there are occasional patients who need colposcopy. These patients have either an abnormality in their Pap smear or a situation in their past gynecological history which requires more significant follow-up than just a Pap smear. I refer these patients to a gynecologist who, because of the nature of his practice, needs to perform colposcopy on a daily basis. Gynecologists or groups of gynecologists with practices large enough to legitimately require colposcopy several times weekly could properly perform their own procedures. But some gynecologists who select their patients properly would probably not use it often enough to acquire the necessary expertise.

The problem with ultrasound equipment is much more serious because other factors are involved. Colposcopy is obviously a harmless procedure. Whether ultrasound is harmless remains to be seen.

The ultrasound instrument utilizes sound waves to create a picture of structures within the body. High-frequency sound waves are passed through soft tissue until they reach tissue of different acoustic density. They are reflected back, reconverted to an electrical signal, and displayed on the screen of an oscilloscope. The value of ultrasound equipment to obstetricians is phenomenal. It can locate the position of the placenta with great accuracy, can give us a definitive dating of the length of the pregnancy, and can even identify some congenital abnormalities!

Ultrasound equipment can also perform in less significant ways. With some degree of accuracy, it can be used to determine the baby's sex before birth. It can even be watched as a "motion picture" of the baby swimming around in the uterus. But these functions can involve abuses. Some physicians perform ultrasound on *every one* of their patients. Some even do the test repeatedly on each patient. While the care of many patients can be enhanced with ultrasound testing (I test about 20 percent), the remainder are merely being given access to a new "toy." The naked truth is that some doctors are using ultrasound as a device to attract patients to their offices by providing them with more fun during pregnancy.

What's wrong with this? Even if we forget the economic factors involved, we cannot ignore the possibility that some permanent damage may accrue from this unnecessary usage. The long-range impact of ultrasound is unknown. Any harmful effects on the fetus might be delayed and difficult to find. Although none has been found so far in humans, studies in mice have shown adverse effects such as chromosomal changes and lowered birth weight.

Neither the mechanism of ultrasound's effects nor the acoustic properties of human tissue is understood well enough to know whether these effects in mice have any significance to humans. Moreover, the mouse experiments were done with ultrasound dosage higher than that used in diagnostic studies. If humans are adversely affected by ultrasound, the effects are certainly not obvious at this time.

At a recent symposium at Columbia University's College of Physicians and Surgeons, Dr. Doreen Leibeskind of the Albert Einstein College of Medicine in New York recommended avoiding frivolous use of ultrasound, saying, "If we err on the side of caution, we'll have no cause for regret." In an even more pointed statement, Dr. Frederick W. Krembau, Associate Professor of Diagnostic Radiology at Yale University School of Medicine, advised, "Don't use ultrasound for fun or to watch the baby." The American College of Radiology and National Institutes of Health (NIH) have also urged that ultrasound be used only when *medically* indicated.

A recent report by an NIH expert panel included the following as medical reasons to do ultrasound:

- Estimation of fetal age in cases where this is clinically uncertain but important to know—for example, if cesarean section, termination of pregnancy, or induction of labor must be appropriately scheduled
- Evaluation of fetal growth in cases of suspected disease
- Vaginal bleeding of undetermined cause
- Determination of fetal position
- Suspected multiple gestation
- Suspected ectopic pregnancy
- Significant discrepancy between size of uterus and estimated stage of pregnancy
- Pelvic mass
- Suspected congenital defect
- As an adjunct to amniocentesis.

The panelists suggested that women ask their doctors: "Why do I need this exam? What would we learn from it? And what benefit can I expect from it?"

I can recall quite vividly the fun I had as a child when my mother took me to the shoe store. How I loved the great big box under which I could put my feet. Through the x-ray machine I could see the bones of my toes inside my shoes! It was marvelous! I could not do it enough! How frightening that is today in light of what we know about the long-range effects of x-rays. X-ray examinations should be done only when the medical advantages outweigh the possible risks. The same policy should be followed for ultrasound. Nobody knows whether ultrasound will ultimately be discovered to be dangerous to the fetus. Where there is a clear medical reason to use it, there is no reason to worry about "possible unknown effects." But until ultrasound is proven completely harmless, there is no justification for using it as a toy.

Like the colposcope, ultrasound should be in the hands of physicians who find the need to use it on a frequent basis. In most communities, this will be the radiologists, a large obstetrical group, or occasionally an obstetrician who specializes in high-risk pregnancies. For both medical and economic reasons it certainly ought not be owned by every obstetrician.

Laboratory machinations

Many physicians obtain blood specimens in their offices and send them to outside laboratories for diagnostic testing. Whether doctors should profit from this procedure has been the subject of considerable controversy in recent years.

The usual set-up is as follows. The laboratory supplies the physician—free-of-charge—with test-tubes, syringes, a centrifuge, and other equipment needed to obtain and prepare the blood samples for testing. (The centrifuge, which costs several hundred dollars, is used to separate blood cells from serum so that they can be tested separately.) The specimens are picked up at the doctor's office once daily and test reports are delivered on the following day. (Abnormal findings with urgent significance are telephoned to the doctor as soon as discovered.) The laboratory gives its physician-clients a price list which enables the doctor to set a fee for each procedure. The doctor collects from the individual patients and pays the lab once a month.

In theory, this is an efficient and economical process for both doctor and patient. Patients are spared the bother of having to travel to another location to provide the specimen, and doctors who choose to do so can make a modest profit even if they charge patients less than they would pay at hospitals and independent laboratories. In practice, however, this system can be subject to abuse. Doctors who perform unnecessary tests or who charge much more than the lab charges them can make considerable profit.

Many lawmakers and insurance companies believe that doctors should not be allowed to profit from testing performed outside of their offices. One proposed solution is a law that forbids billing by someone who doesn't actually perform the service. Doctors could charge a fee for drawing and processing the blood specimens, but patients or insurance companies would pay the labs directly. Insurance companies would pay fees similar to those charged to doctors, but patients paying the lab directly would pay "retail" prices. This set-up would prevent abuses by the small number of doctors who might wish to take advantage of the system. But it would also raise the overhead of the outside labs, who, in turn, would raise their prices to the public.

When a doctor refers a patient to a commercial laboratory for testing, the usual procedure is that the laboratory obtains the specimen to be tested and collects its fee either from the patient or the patient's insurance company. However, some laboratories are willing to bill the referring doctor who charges the patient a higher fee and thereby makes a profit. This is different from the set-up where the doctor's office obtains the specimen and prepares it for the lab.

There is some labor involved in obtaining and preparing the specimen in a doctor's office. But in the referral method, the doctor's staff does virtually nothing. Some doctors rationalize that they are entitled to a fee for interpreting the test, but interpreting a lab test usually takes only a few seconds. Do you think that doctors should be entitled to profit in this situation? Do you think that a doctor who does so might be tempted to choose the lab which offers the highest kickback rather than the one which does the highest quality work? Do you think that doctors who profit in this manner will be tempted to order unnecessary tests? I don't know how many doctors use (or abuse) such set-ups, but the New York State legislature thought the situation sufficiently out-of-hand that it passed a law stating that only the provider who performs a service (obtains the specimen or carries out the test) may bill the patient.

Obstetricians and gynecologists do not usually need to order as many outpatient lab tests as some other physicians do (particularly general practitioners and internists who treat a wider range of diseases), so few of them participate in the abuses described above.

The ideal system for laboratory testing would be for doctors to obtain specimens in their offices, order tests only when needed, and make only a reasonable profit from the tests. While laws or insurance regulations can stop some abuses, they may also raise costs for some of the patients of ethical physicians. Your best protection from "laboratory abuse" is to select your physician with care. If you expect to have a considerable amount of laboratory testing, you might compare the price of lab tests done in the doctor's office with those done in hospital and independent laboratories. If you think a doctor is making too much on tests, you can ask to see his laboratory pricelist. If a doctor refers you to a commercial laboratory but collects the fee in his office, something unethical or even illegal may be taking place.

8

PRUDENT BREAST MANAGEMENT

There is probably no disease more frightening to women than breast cancer. There is good reason for this: breast malignancy occurs in 1 out of 11 women in our population and accounts for 27 percent of all malignancies in women. It is almost 400 times as common as vaginal cancer following DES usage. *There is no malignancy in women more prevalent than breast cancer.*

Over the years, there has been little progress in improving survival rates for women within any particular stage of the malignancy. Thus the best way to improve survival rates lies in earlier detection. Of the many methods of tumor detection that have been studied, an appropriate combination of self-examination, periodic examination by a physician, and mammography appears to yield the most satisfactory results. However, at a national conference sponsored by the American College of Radiology in 1982, several speakers indicated that many physicians were either not performing breast examinations or doing them in a cursory manner.

Dr. Gordon F. Schwartz of Jefferson Medical College, Philadelphia, indicated that since the advent of mammography, thorough and complete physical examinations of the breast have taken a back seat. The same may be said for taking an adequate history. Women who have not breast-fed and those who have a family history of breast cancer have an increased risk of developing the disease. But, Dr. Schwartz noted, many doctors fail to obtain this information from their patients. In another presentation, Dr. Loren J. Humphrey stated that teaching women how to examine their own breasts is the "single best thing we can do for them."

Breast self-examination (BSE)

Four out of five breast malignancies are first identified by patients and subsequently called to the doctor's attention; only one out of five is discovered by a physician. In contrast to cervical cancer for which a yearly checkup is certainly sufficient, checking the breasts once a year is just as certainly *not* sufficient. Pap smears can detect premalignant changes several years before cancer appears. But the danger of breast cancer is not detectable until cancer is actually present.

One of the largest studies of breast self-examination appeared in the journal *Cancer* in 1981. Drs. Huguley and Brown of the Emory University School of Medicine in Atlanta, Georgia, who evaluated more than 2,000 women with breast cancer, found that two-thirds of them had practiced some form of BSE, although only half of them did it every month as recommended by the American Cancer Society.

The stage of the disease at the time of discovery was related to whether or not the women did BSE. Of those doing BSE, 85 percent discovered their disease while it was still in a favorable stage for treatment. In nonexamining patients, only 62 percent of the cancers were in favorable stages. Other researchers have reported similar findings. Obviously, BSE increases the likelihood of discovering breast cancers while they are still treatable.

The Atlanta study found that women who learned BSE from a physician or nurse rather than from publications, television, or American Cancer Society training sessions were more likely to perform the procedure monthly. Some doctors provide this training diligently, some in a cursory manner, and some not at all. Most gynecologists urge their patients to have a Pap smear annually (or more often) to detect cervical cancer, a disease much less common than breast cancer. Yet some do not take the time to promote breast self-examination and train their patients in its technique.

A recent survey by the National Cancer Institute indicated that 77 percent of adult females did some form of BSE but only 29 percent did it monthly.

Several reasons are given by women for not performing breast self-examination. Prominent among them are fears of either "finding something" or of overlooking a significant problem. Overcoming these worries can require a great deal of time, patience and understanding from the physician. The doctors should attempt to persuade their anxious patients that this type of care should *relieve* some of their anxiety by giving them a much better chance of survival should they unfortunately be affected. There is no way to guarantee that any individual will not be the unfortunate target of breast cancer. We can only strive to recognize it early and conquer it with the means we have at hand.

The second worry mentioned above should be much easier to overcome. This problem results from the *mistaken* assumption that women should be capable of identifying breast cancer. That is, in fact, not the goal of BSE; its purpose is to help patients learn what their breasts feel like. Breasts vary considerably from woman to woman. Some are free of lumps while others are quite cystic. Women who check their breasts unfailingly month after month will learn to recognize if a *change* has occurred. If a change is detected, a doctor can evaluate its significance.

Women who rely completely on their doctors for breast checks are asking for trouble. Without self-examination, too much time may pass between checks. That, of course, would be true even if all doctors did careful breast examinations. But many don't. Without thorough examinations, many cancers won't be detected until it is too late to save the patient.

The following is the method of self-examination recommended by the American Cancer Society.

There are two basic steps. The easiest is the mirror check. First look at your breasts in the mirror with your arms at your side. Raise your arms over your head to see if either breast shows any unusual change in size or shape. Also put your hands on your hips, press down, and see if you notice anything different. See if there are changes in the skin, or any redness, swelling, sore, or scaly area on the nipple.

The second step takes longer to explain than to do. Lie down on your back on a bed or other flat surface. Place a small pillow or folded towel under your right shoulder and put your right arm behind your head. Use your left hand to check the right breast. Keep your fingers flat and together. Think of your breast as the face of a clock. Start at 12 o'clock and gently press around till you're back up to 12 again. You must cover every part of the breast. When you've finished put the pillow under your left shoulder, your left arm behind your head, and use your right hand to check your left breast. Simple. Then gently squeeze each nipple to see whether a discharge is produced.

The breast should be checked once a month. The best time is after a menstrual period, when hormonal activity is at its lowest ebb. Women who are no longer menstruating should select a time for BSE that is easy to remember, such as the first of each month. Some authorities recommend a "wet exam," done in the shower, as part of the technique. Wetness apparently increases the ability to detect minor changes in breast tissue.

A lump that enlarges, a dominant mass, an increase in the size or consistency of one breast, changes in the skin of the nipple, or nipple discharge should be reported to one's physician. Incidentally, breast pain and tenderness, especially if they occur in both breasts, are usually *not* signs of malignancy.

Mammography

Mammography is a procedure for using x-rays to examine the female breast for cancer. In 1983, the American Cancer Society endorsed 1982 guidelines published by the American College of Radiology calling for: 1) a baseline mammogram between the ages of 35 and 40; 2) mammograms every year or two from 40 to 49; and 3) annual mammograms from age 50 and over.

Both medical and lay literature are being bombarded by opinions about the use of mammography as possibly the most effective tool in identifying breast malignancies in the earliest stages (under 2 centimeters in diameter). There is some risk involved in having an annual x-ray examination, but recent improvements in mammography have resulted in much lower radiation doses and better detection ability. Much research is being done, and it appears likely that mammography will become the definitive procedure for early diagnosis.

If mammography shows that a mass does not appear cancerous, surgery may be avoided. However, suspicious lumps may still need removal even if the mammography study is normal.

Benign breast lumps

Many different terms are used to describe the findings from breast examinations. Some of these can be confusing or even sound ominous. The term "fibrocystic disease" is the most widely used and has become a general term for all sorts of breast abnormalities. Fibrocystic disease is most common in women over age 25 and tends to improve after menopause. The condition is actually an over-response of breast tissue to hormonal stimulation. It is characterized by pain, tenderness and lumpiness that may increase prior to menstrual periods and decrease afterwards. The incidence of cancer in women with fibrocystic disease is slightly higher than in women who have no breast abnormalities. The major problem in medical management is to be sure that a cancer present in fibrocystic breasts is not overlooked.

A second type of benign lump is the fibroadenoma, typically found in women in their teens and twenties. It is a smooth, solitary, highly movable mass with a rubbery consistency. In most cases, the appropriate treatment is simply periodic re-examination of the patient.

A third, less common type of benign tumor is the

intraductal papilloma. This typically presents with a nipple discharge and can be felt as a small nodule near the edge of the nipple. The usual treatment is surgical removal through a small cosmetic incision around the nipple.

Management of breast lumps

The management of patients with breast lumps is not without its problems. I feel somewhat wary about presenting this information, for it certainly does not fall into the same category as the unnecessary hysterectomy. As noted in Chapter 3, some doctors exaggerate the risk of uterine cancer to promote hysterectomies. When tumors are found in the uterus, they are almost always benign (noncancerous) fibroids that need no surgery whatsoever.

In the case of breast cancer, however, not only is the risk high, but often it is quite difficult to make an accurate judgment based on the examination alone. Yet surgery should not be done every time a breast lump appears! There is probably no woman who will not have a breast lump at some time in her life. By far the great majority of these lumps will be benign. What is a rational approach?

The answer lies in attempting through nonsurgical means to make the best possible judgments about when the surgery is advisable. The first step should be a thorough history and physical exam. The physical exam should check not only the lumpy area, but both breasts completely.

If the lump feels cystic (a cyst is a fluid-filled sac), one possible approach is to attempt to withdraw the fluid. If fluid is obtained, if it is clear (not bloody or brownish) and contains no malignant cells when viewed under the microscope, no surgery need be performed.

If the lesion is solid but appears benign to the physician, and the patient is under 35 years of age, probably nothing should be done except to reassure the patient and arrange to check the lump again in about three months. BSE should, of course, be performed monthly during the interim. If the patient is over 35 and fluid cannot be aspirated, mammography should be performed. If the mam-

Table 8:1. Management of Breast Lumps

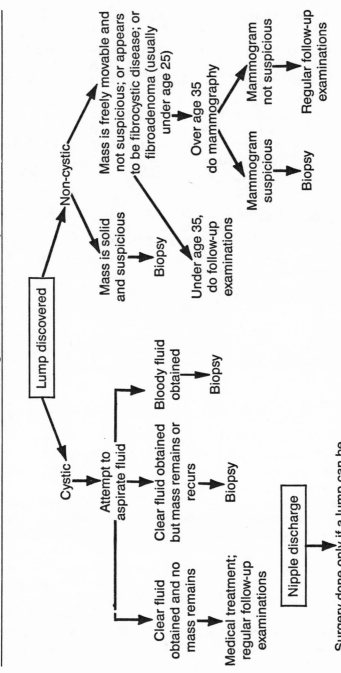

mographic study is normal, follow-up exams should be scheduled as noted above. However, if the mammogram looks suspicious, a biopsy should be performed even if the lesion feels benign. Similarly, if the lesion feels suspicious, biopsy should be performed even if mammography is normal.

When a biopsy confirms a diagnosis of benign fibrocystic disease, a number of non-surgical approaches can be tried. Among these are caffeine restriction, hormonal treatment, dietary treatment, and diuretics.

This overall strategy is summarized in Table 8:1.

Trouble in Texas

My research makes it clear that many doctors are too quick to operate. Table 8:2 shows what happened to patients who had breast biopsies at a hospital in Texas during a recent 1-year period.

Table 8:2. Outcome of Breast Biopsies

Patient Age	No. Patients	No. Cancers	% with Cancer
Over age 50	134	54	40.3%
Under age 50	82	6	7.3%
Under age 40	88	6	6.8%
Under age 30	44	0	0.0%
All ages combined	348	66	19.0%

This chart should not be interpreted to mean that breast cancer is never seen below age 30. The risk, however, is obviously small.

It was disconcerting to find that although a number of surgeons reported only from 5 to 12 percent of their breast surgery patients under the age of 30, there were some whose operating record revealed 20 percent or more of their cases were done in this low-risk group.

Another piece of statistical information was disturbing. By examining all of the cases for each physician, one could determine what percentage of the biopsies performed were ultimately found to result in a diagnosis of cancer. No specific rate of identifying cancers could be singled out as ideal or expected. But, as shown above, 19 percent of the entire group of biopsies were malignant.

Many surgeons had a much better rate in their selection of cases for biopsy. Some were accurate in their diagnosis over 40 percent of the time, others in the 30s and still more between 20 and 30 percent. There were others, however, in whose cases the rate of malignancy was in the low teens, under 10 percent and even down to zero. Though the diagnosis may be difficult to make, one should wonder about such large discrepancies in accuracy among different physicians.

No one is more frightened than the patient who is told she must have a breast biopsy. It almost never occurs to her to have a second opinion. The surgery is immediately scheduled. Yet there is actually no more logic to going ahead with breast surgery without a second opinion than any other type of operation. All surgeons are very wary of missing a breast malignancy, and none will recommend avoiding surgery when there is even the slightest doubt. Possibly, however, the use of second opinions on all cases would reduce the number of operations on younger, lower risk patients. It also might create more of a balance in the percentage of malignancies seen in each physician's series. If some doctors' judgments are too frequently in error, then possibly a second opinion will stabilize their operative rate. Because of the high risk of breast cancer, patients ought not to decide by themselves that surgery need not be done. But there is no reason why a second opinion should not be sought as described in the final chapter of this book. Doctors certainly don't want to markedly reduce the biopsy rate if this means increasing the number of missed cases. That, however, does not mean that it might not be possible to improve the selection of operative patients.

Conservative care combined with breast self-examination should make it possible to improve the cure rate of breast cancer while at the same time avoiding surgery when the risk of cancer is not high.

9

A TALE OF
TWO HOSPITALS

Previous chapters of this book discuss the surgical rates
for various procedures performed at either of two
hospitals, one in New York and one in Texas. To place this
situation in greater perspective, let's compare the two
hospitals. Hospital A is a community hospital which
enjoys an excellent reputation despite essentially no self-
policing of its surgical procedures. Hospital B is
university-affiliated with a reasonable amount of peer
review, though far from perfect. During the time of the
study, it had the same number of active gynecologists as
Hospital A but approximately two-thirds the number of
deliveries.

Hysterectomies in young women

How many women in their twenties would have an adequate reason to be subjected to a hysterectomy? During my
twenty years of practice I have seen very few. During a
two-year period at Hospital B there were only two. During
just one year at Hospital A there were 82! *It is impossible
for this number to be justifiable.*

Is it possible that Hospital A's doctors treated more
patients or treated younger patients? For either to be the

case, we would expect that the number of deliveries at Hospital A would be vastly greater—perhaps 40 times greater—than that of Hospital B. But this is obviously not the situation. Even if Hospital A's community patient population were 10 times that of Hospital B, its rate of hysterectomies in patients under 30 would not be justified. At Hospital B only 0.65 percent of the hysterectomies were done on women under 30. At Hospital A this figure was 11.3 percent—*17 times as great!* Thirty-five percent of the hysterectomies on women under 30 at Hospital A were done by four (13 percent) of the 30 doctors.

Disgraceful D&Cs

As noted in Chapter 3, dysfunctional or irregular bleeding is almost never an adequate reason to perform a D&C in a woman under age 40. There are occasional reasons for premenopausal women to have this operation, but the number of such women should be small. (D&Cs done for pregnancy-related conditions, i.e., abortion, miscarriage or postpartum bleeding are not included in this discussion.)

The statistics in Chapter 3, collected in Hospital B, demonstrated some improvement when the doctors became aware that they were being observed. During that year, 515 non-pregnancy-related D&Cs were done at Hospital B while Hospital A had 832. At hospital B, 29 percent of these operations were done on women under 40. This number is still too high and indicates that many should not have been done. But at Hospital A, this figure was 53 percent; eight doctors there had rates between 62 and 79 percent and three ranged from 81 to 87 percent!

These rates make my blood boil! Every one of these operations subjected a patient to the risks of general anesthesia. Some of the physicians involved were (and some still are) in positions of authority at their hospital.

Ovarian operations

As noted in Chapter 6, symptomatic ovarian cysts occur commonly in young women during a reproductive cycle.

These usually resolve by themselves within a few weeks and do not require surgery. Ovarian cancer, on the other hand, is rare in women under 40, and when it is present, the diagnosis is usually apparent before the surgery is performed. For these reasons, most ovarian surgery should be performed in women over 40.

At Hospital A, excluding operations for possible tubal pregnancies, sterilization or infertility, there were 246 operations for suspected ovarian disease. Of these, 94 were laparoscopies (in which an instrument is inserted through the abdominal wall to look inside) and 152 were laparotomies (open abdominal operations). Nineteen of the patients were teenagers, 127 were in their twenties, 70 were in their thirties, and only 30 were above age 40. Seven doctors were responsible for 37 percent of these operations. Seventy-six percent of their patients were in their teens and twenties.

Ectopic pregnancies

Data on ectopic pregnancies are available only from Hospital A, but the comparison between doctors will suffice. There were 34 ectopic pregnancies identified and operated upon in 1980. Some of these were fairly obvious before the surgery was begun and some were uncertain until the abdomen was entered. During the same year there were 40 operative procedures recorded for "possible ectopic pregnancy" which found no such condition, and only a few cases had another condition serious enough to require surgery. There will always be a few cases in which the diagnosis is sufficiently difficult to make that surgery appropriate even when it reveals no serious condition. But this should not happen in more than half the cases!

The accuracy rate of some doctors at Hospital A was excellent in determining whether surgery was necessary. Two doctors who did four operations each were correct 75 percent of the time, while several others who performed three or less were 100 percent accurate. However, those who operated the most had accuracy rates of 20 percent (1 in 5), 14 percent (1 in 7) and 25 percent (3 in 12).

Cutting the hymen

There was a time in gynecology when women came to their physicians and related that they were unable to have intercourse because their husbands could not enter through their hymenal ring. In the past—the distant past—they were taken to the operating room so that the hymen could be cut open. Then it was discovered that painful scar tissue often formed where the cut was made. Now it is generally accepted that these women can be taught to gently stretch the vaginal opening by hand, until they reach a point where further stretching can be achieved by loving and tender intercourse. It has been more than 20 years since I did one of these operations.

At Hospital B, hymenectomy was performed only once during 1981. At Hospital A, however, this procedure was done 6 times—all by two doctors. Twenty-eight gynecologists did not do one single case of that type during the entire year. Had those six patients obtained a second opinion, would those operations have been scheduled? I think not.

Primary C-section rates

As noted in Chapter 5, the primary C-section rates at Hospital A were 13.8 percent in 1981 and 19.7 percent in 1983. The comparable figures for Hospital B were 12 and 15 percent, far from perfect, but considerably lower. In 1977, the last year I was Director of Obstetrics and Gynecology at Hospital B, the rate was only 7 percent!

The role of the hospital

It is apparent that Hospital A, which has virtually no peer review, compares unfavorably to Hospital B for every type of surgery evaluated in this book. Table 9:1 demonstrates this and illustrates the statistics of the six worst offenders on the staff of Hospital A.

Abuses are most frequent in hospitals where unethical physicians control most of what goes on, where administration and boards of directors are weak or look the other

Table 9:1. Questionable surgical rates
(Percentages rounded to nearest whole number)

	Hysterectomy on patients under 30 (%)	D&C under age 40 (%)	Ovarian exploration under age 40 (%)	Primary C-section rate (%) 1981	Primary C-section rate (%) 1983	Hymenectomy (number done)
Hospital B (University-affiliated)	1%	29%	Not available	12%	15%	1
Hospital A (Community hospital)	11%	53%	88%	14%	20%	6
Dr. P	33%	50%	100%			
Dr. Q	22%	87%	100%			
Dr. R	18%	18%	100%			
Dr. S	10%	81%	100%			
Dr. T	18%	81%	71%			
Dr. U	15%	70%	83%			

way. In big cities where economic pressures are greatest, abuses are often rampant except in hospitals affiliated with medical schools. Surveillance tends to be best in teaching hospitals, but there is no guarantee that it is effective. The only hospitals in which substantial protection exists are those where highly motivated physicians in positions of power are determined to regulate what happens. When no control exists, unethical gynecologists can run roughshod over their patient population.

When I reviewed all the work in the Ob/Gyn department of Hospital A, it was obvious that the doctors with the highest rates of inappropriate surgery for one procedure were unethical in other areas. They did the greatest numbers of D&Cs on all ages. They operated more and performed more hysterectomies on young women than their peers did. They were also involved in overutilization of nonsurgical procedures.

At a meeting of a Gynecology Department I attended, a surgical case was presented in which the need for surgery was questioned. Dr. T stood up to defend his fellow physician's decision to operate. He stated that he had a similar patient who had been seen by two other gynecologists who had refused to perform a hysterectomy on her. In fact, they had already looked into her abdomen with a laparoscope and determined that there was no gynecological pathology. Undaunted, Dr. T indicated that he was planning to do a hysterectomy anyway. When confronted with "What would be the indication for such surgery?" and "What is your diagnosis?" his response was, "Oh! I'll find something!"

Are there a small number of Dr. T's at every hospital? How many hospitals won't tolerate their unethical behavior? At one hospital where I once served, an effort was made in that direction. But even there, it was only when the physician's unnecessary surgery resulted in complications. Remember that physicians who abuse with skilled hands almost never get them slapped.

The ultimate absurdity

As a final touch to this chapter, I'd like to tell you about the most outlandish abuse I have seen. Chapter 4 points out that when vaginal hysterectomy is done, the diagnosis is almost always uterine prolapse (the uterus dropping down through the vagina)—but that hysterectomy for slight prolapse is rarely appropriate. Conversely, when prolapse is severe enough to warrant hysterectomy, the safest and most sensible way to remove the uterus is vaginally.

At Hospital A, 15 cases disgnosed as uterine prolapse were treated by *abdominal* hysterectomy. The obvious explanation is that in these cases the patient's uterus had not dropped sufficiently to enable the surgeon to remove it vaginally! That diagnosis was used—in the absence of disease—because no other diagnosis could be faked! How ridiculous and deceitful.

10

UNDERSTANDING
AN UNHEALTHY
MEDICAL WORLD

M ost of this book describes problems for which doctors are responsible—either individually or collectively. This chapter examines some additional problems which aggravate the situation but cannot be solved by doctors alone.

The doctor surplus

Although there is good reason to believe that our health care system offers the best care and the best physicians in the world, the advances in medicine have been available primarily to the urban middle class and to the wealthy. The primary goal of policymakers in the field of medical sociology has been to make the advantages of our medical system available to all our citizens. That includes proper care for those who live in the less advantaged areas of our cities as well as those in rural America.

It was hoped that training physicians from lower economic groups would increase the number and quality of physicians practicing in the lower economic ghettos. But black or Hispanic doctors turned out to be no more interested in serving black or Hispanic slums than white doctors have been interested in serving white slums. So, although it was proper for medical schools to become more liberal and to select more minority students, this did not solve the problems of delivering medical care to the poor.

It was also thought that if the number of physicians were increased, doctors would spread out more into rural areas. Medical schools increase their output greatly, but recent graduates were no more eager to move into rural areas than were the doctors who preceded them. Moreover, many urban areas have become supersaturated with doctors, particularly specialists.

Increased utilization

It is common knowledge that when the supply of a product becomes greater than the demand for it, competition drives prices down. However, this does not seem to apply to medical practice! Medical care is not something people can do without. Patients are essentially a captive audience in a market where suppliers set prices which are usually fairly uniform in a given community. Most physicians set their fees by estimating how much money they want to make and the number of patients they expect to see. If the demand for their services is low, most doctors tend to charge higher fees.

Even more distressing, income can also be increased by performing unnecessary services. As demonstrated throughout this book, some doctors have been doing exactly that. So our society's efforts to improve the level of medical care by increasing the number of physicians, though well intended, have created problems for many patients. The number of medical students is now being reduced, but it will take many years for the surplus of physicians to be relieved.

Government controls?

In recent years, medical costs have been skyrocketing. Some people think this problem should be attacked by increasing government control over medical practice. But this approach, like the ones discussed above, may create more problems than it solves. This can be seen by examining some current types of government-controlled programs.

In England, where medicine has been socialized for many years, a great portion of the populace is quite pleased at receiving its care without concern for its cost. The fear of massive individual expenditures has been eliminated. Even the concern over moderate costs, which at times limits Americans from getting any care, is not a restricting factor in England. Patients there have no qualms about seeking medical advice for even the most minor problems. The result is that their facilities are overcrowded. The demand for necessary but elective surgery so far exceeds the available facilities that the waiting time can sometimes stretch into years. Physicians earning fixed incomes are not inclined to work overtime to eliminate such long waiting periods, but some doctors run private practices that cater to patients willing to pay high fees for prompter and more personalized care.

Care at government facilities in America is also quite variable. Centers such as Walter Reed Hospital and Brooke Army Hospital offer outstanding care. However, most military medical care is administered at smaller facilities run by physicians with little drive or initiative. Veterans Administration hospitals affiliated with teaching institutions or medical centers are like the best military installations; doctors who are highly motivated and research-oriented provide fine care. But at lower levels, the care is provided by physicians with less motivation and probably less technical ability, who could not attain positions in the finer installations or be successful in private practice.

At crowded clinics, military facilities and veterans hospitals, many patients wait inordinate lengths of time to see a physician. The attitudes of nurses and other employees are often very impersonal. There may be little or no concern about important emotional or psychological problems related to the illness. Where an emotional component has not preceded the illness, it may certainly become a factor to the patient who feels like a number.

Some physicians in these situations are highly motivated to accomplish something worthwhile for their patients and for medical science in general. Unfortunately, others are primarily interested in having a position with little responsibility, 9-to-5 hours, and none of the pressures of private practice. In many cases, the physician claims as a basis for his choice a more healthy family life of his own. However, the net result is often insufficient concern about whether the patient is seen today or tomorrow.

The Medicaid program was conceived in an effort to bring better medical care to the needy through private care subsidized by federal and state governments. However, two factors make it almost impossible for ethical private physicians to participate in the program in any major way. Fee schedules are far below standard fees, and payment is often extremely slow. Paperwork commonly must go back and forth several times, with the secretarial expense ending up greater than the ultimate payment.

Most physicians, even those who believe that it is socially responsible to participate in the Medicaid program, find it economically suicidal to do so. But a number of doctors have developed ways to deal with Medicaid unethically. Through all sorts of maneuvers, they manipulate the system to earn a considerable amount of money. A few physicians have large but honest Medicaid practices, but almost all reputable and ethical doctors can afford to treat only a smattering of such patients.

Problems at training centers

So far I have talked about problems related to overutilization motivated by money. Overutilization can also occur for other reasons in some of the best public institutions—where interns, residents and fellows are trained. In their zeal to learn all they possibly can, there is the tendency for doctors in postgraduate training to subject patients to surgery which might otherwise be avoided. The medical problems are usually those that might properly be handled in more than one way, but the surgical approach is selected for training purposes.

Unfortunately, even in the finest training centers,

insufficient effort appears to be devoted to medical ethics. That defect was painfully obvious in a recent conversation I had with a senior resident at a major teaching institution. He told me that his opportunity to perform surgery depended upon the frequency with which he could operate with private gynecologists in the community. Those who operated the most were doing many unnecessary cases. He decided that if he questioned them about case selection, they would stop allowing him to operate with them. Since he felt that his questioning would have no effect on their ethics and yet have a negative effect on his training, he decided to remain silent. I could not help but wonder whether he or his fellow trainees were being corrupted.

Underutilization

It has been proposed that unnecessary surgery could be curtailed by placing all surgeons on salaries. The rate of surgery would no doubt be reduced, but other problems would certainly occur.

In 1979, a very important research project was released which dealt with the rates of surgery under two types of prepaid insurance programs in Seattle, Washington. Under one plan, doctors in a large group were salaried and therefore had no financial incentive to do surgery. In the other program, doctors in independent practice were paid on a fee-for-service basis.

The study, which took years to complete, involved reviewing the charts of those in both plans who underwent hysterectomy, removal of tonsils and/or adenoids, appendectomy, and gallbladder surgery. Using a complex system of evaluation, a panel of physicians judged whether the operations were necessary, appropriate or justifiable. Then the figures were carefully analyzed to allow for differences in the size of the groups and the sex and ages of the patients. As seen in other studies, there was a significant rate of inappropriate selection in the fee-for-service cases. The panel judged that 21 percent of the hysterectomies done by fee-for-service doctors were not justified. But they also found that fee-for-service physicians performed almost seven times as many *justified* hysterectomies as their prepaid colleagues—which suggests that where there are no financial incentives, physicians may not recommend all the operations which *are* justifiable!

Like all other individuals who have incentives removed from their occupations, physicians tend to lose enthusiasm for achieving the highest levels in their professional performance. As much as we would wish otherwise, personal pride is not a sufficient driving force for most people. The most satisfactory results in every segment of society are seen where people are encouraged to improve themselves by the use of incentives. Sometimes those incentives relate to status, but much more frequently they are economic. Even countries whose official beliefs reject that concept have at times wavered and allowed such incentives to exist in order to save their faltering economies.

Medical realities

If answers to our problems are to be found, it will be necessary for us to be realistic in assessing what these problems are. It is important that we honestly face the truth that both private and public medicine today has serious flaws.

Continued abuse by some private practice physicians, unrestricted in any way by the remainder of the profession, may impel our government to seize control of medical practice. But examination of current government-controlled programs makes me believe that this would be disastrous for both the public and the medical profession.

For our democratic society to survive, government must be involved in some way to provide for those who are needy. There are no simple or pat solutions. But our society should strive to provide services with a minimum amount of government involvement. A system which provides the best possible medical care must be multifaceted and flexible. It must acknowledge that incentives are required for physicians to produce the best services. It must realize that greed exists but can be recognized and controlled. It must encourage and demand the highest possible standards of care. Whatever system is created must be modified continually to adjust for changes and new insights.

Above all, one fact should not be overlooked: the cornerstone of medical practice is the doctor-patient relationship. It is clear that the outcome of treatment often depends upon how the patient feels toward the doctor. A system based solely on cost-saving, but which discards human factors, would be a tragic mistake.

There is nothing patients can do about the oversupply of physicians and the policies that contribute to this problem. How then can patients strive for the best possible medical care, the least amount of abuse, and reasonable fees? Even more important, how can patients form trusting relationships with their doctors? These topics are discussed in the following chapter.

11

HOW TO PROTECT YOURSELF

Physicians have held a special position in our society—but I'm not sure whether this is more good than bad. I do know that because of this position, physicians can inspire confidence which may help patients to overcome some of their ailments more quickly. Thus patients expect that what will be done by their doctor is going to help them. Ultimately, that expectation has to be an important part of medical care which certainly should not be lost.

But what else does that devotion and admiration cause? Does it inspire some physicians to feel God-like? I'm certain that's true. In the past, gynecologists have been almost exclusively male. Recent literature reveals that some of these men have dealt in an extremely sexist manner with their patients. Claims are even made that some of these physicians truly dislike women!

Has that God-like position also created an atmosphere in which patients not only are afraid to question their physician, but in fact, may be chastised or caused to feel guilty if they attempt such an action?

When these kinds of questions are brought up, one must wonder if there is any place for blind trust. Is distrust the only alternative to blind trust? Some commentators would have us believe that.

An active role is needed

It seems to me that the patient's approach should be somewhere between these two unpleasant extremes. Ought not the relationship between physician and patient be one where the patient has great confidence that her doctor will do what is best for her? Yet at the same time, when major decisions are to be made, shouldn't they result from clear and open discussion about the logic and merit of such treatment? Shouldn't patients be told everything there is to know so they can share in the decision-making process? Finally, what makes seeking another opinion a sign of distrust or disloyalty? There is no sense to that kind of thought process. Yet many—perhaps most—physicians feel that way. That type of response can only be blamed on the excessive adulation received by the doctor, leading to massive growth of his ego and an inability to accept the possibility of imperfection. To paraphrase a well known quotation, "Let him who has never made a mistake in medicine be the one to operate without question."

Having relationships of mutual respect with patients has been wonderful for me. It is not just another aspect to my profession; it is an integral part of my life. Physicians are among the few individuals who have the good fortune to spend their working day with people who look to them with trust for advice and counsel. It is indeed a constant ego boost and reinforcement. And for that, there is an obligation to give our patients the best of ourselves.

Unfortunately, it is clear that a small percentage of doctors are grossly abusing the public, and that a much larger percentage make occasional poor judgments. There are five things you can do to protect yourself as a patient:

1) Select your doctors carefully
2) Become well informed
3) Take an active role in your care
4) Don't be afraid to ask for second opinions
5) Press for effective hospital peer review in your community.

Choosing a doctor

Many consumers take less care in making that choice than in almost any other area of life they deal with. They hear a name, or they get sent to see a specific physician and automatically assume that they "belong" to that doctor. Little or no effort may be made to select wisely, to determine whether there is another physician who would better satisfy their needs.

If one is to use a primary care physician—a family practitioner, an internist, a pediatrician or a gynecologist—for most medical problems, doesn't it make sense to spend a few hours making that choice? That doctor may handle crisis situations for a major portion of a human being's life. If a woman is going through the experience of having a baby at most a few times in her life, shouldn't she take the time and effort to be certain of getting the best care possible?

When making the initial selection of a physician, several approaches may be utilized. If you have any friends in the profession, ask them for recommendations or for their opinions of the several doctors you are considering. If you have the time and inclination, make an effort to speak to nurses in the hospitals where the doctors you are considering practice. It is likely that a call to the County Medical Society will only yield a list of names selected at random without any knowledge of the quality of care. So it may be worthwhile to ask other friends whom they use. However, be aware that their information may not be valid either, since their selections may have been made without good basis.

You may want to know whether the doctor you have selected is affiliated with a medical school or hospital that trains interns and residents. It is not essential that your doctor have such affiliations, but it certainly is favorable. If he or she is affiliated with only a small proprietary hospital—unless there is nothing else in your area—that fact would be less favorable.

In choosing an obstetrician/gynecologist, other positive

indicators would be certification by the American Board of Obstetrics and Gynecology and Fellowship in the American College of Obstetrics and Gynecology and/or the American College of Surgeons. However, membership in all of these bodies is still not a guarantee that you will receive the care to which you feel entitled.

Getting acquainted

Most people who buy cars visit several dealers before making their decision. Wouldn't it be sensible to put as much effort into choosing a physician before illness occurs? Making an interview visit before illness or at the onset of pregnancy makes a great deal of sense.

As an example, if a woman is seeking a gynecologist, she might ask many of the following questions:

1. How often will it be necessary for her to be seen?

2. How often should she have a Pap smear?

3. Will the doctor discuss her treatment with her on each visit in the consultation room where they may talk without pressure while she is dressed and more at ease, rather than undressed in the examining room?

4. Can she discuss any sexual problems with the doctor should they arise?

5. Is it possible to call and speak to the doctor either during or after office hours?

6. What are the office fees?

7. Should she expect to have long waiting times in his office?

8. What are the doctor's positions on contraception, abortion, hysterectomy, etc.?

Obviously, the best thing that can happen is for a woman to find a wonderful doctor to whom she can relate beautifully. That trusting relationship will serve to benefit both doctor and patient. However, that expectation may not come to fruition and it is urgent that the selection of a physician not be irrevocable. If a patient seems to feel uncomfortable in some way, she should continue to seek out someone who gives her a reason to develop confidence. Sometimes that will be impossible because it is the patient who is incapable of establishing such a relationship. But most of the time, the diligent patient will find that doctor who provides the care and psychological nourishment necessary for her well-being.

Become informed

Probably the most important concept to maintain throughout this relation is whether there is free-flowing communication between doctor and patient. The patient should recognize that something is wrong if her doctor is using phrases like "trust me," "I know what's best for you," or "It's best for you to let me make the decision on this matter." *If a patient does not feel involved in the decision-making process, she is probably in the wrong place.* That is not to say that the doctor ought not to be giving advice to the patient. It means that when he makes his recommendation, it should be accompanied by an explanation so that the patient understands the reason for the treatment.

Patient responsibility

Patients, too, have certain obligations. The burden must fall on you as consumers of medical care to help solve many of the problems presented in this book. Being well-informed and taking an active role in your care involves learning about your condition. Libraries and public service organizations generally have a good deal of literature available that can help you become knowledgeable about the symptoms and suggested methods of treatment. (An excellent book—though I disagree with a few of its details—is *The Complete Guide to Women's Health*, by Bruce D. Shephard, M.D., and Caroll A. Shephard, R.N., Ph.D., published in 1982 by Mariner Publishing Co., Tampa, Florida.) With that information in hand, you can have an intelligent and logical discussion with your doctor about the proposed treatment.

Don't forget that aside from the many minor errors that may occur we have referred to the possibility of two million unnecessary operations annually! Does it boggle your mind to realize that this number means 1 unneeded operation every 16 seconds? I have made it clear throughout this book that a major part of the responsibility for this will have to fall on the patient. It is possible for a questioning public to make significant improvements in all of the areas we have delved into.

Second opinions

In major decisions, such as whether surgery should be performed, the method of handling such choices is much clearer. *IT IS ALMOST NEVER ADVISABLE TO UNDERGO NON-EMERGENCY SURGERY WITHOUT ANOTHER OPINION.* That second opinion should be sought at a location some distance away from the initial physician. If one lives in a large city, the consultation should be with a doctor who has no relationship with your own physician. If you live in a small community with only a few gynecologists, you will probably be best served by getting another opinion from a doctor in another city. The importance of accomplishing that will be well worth the cost.

If you have good insurance coverage, the cost of that second opinion will be paid by the company, and wisely so. The company will probably even select the consulting physician. If, however, it is necessary to find your own consultant, then other techniques may be utilized. Referrals can be sought from medical schools or highly recommended physicians.

When seeking the opinion, certain ground rules should be followed. The consultant should be honestly told the reason for the visit. It is probably better not to reveal the name of your physician until after the consultation has been completed. It should be understood *absolutely* from the very beginning that the consultant will serve only to offer an opinion as to the best available treatment. Under no circumstances should he or she be involved in the treatment. No matter how much the consulting physician may impress you, this doctor should never be permitted to become the operating physician. The very possibility of that occurring will eliminate the most important characteristic of the consultation—objectivity.

If, after having that consultation, the patient finds that she is in a position where the two opinions differ, it may be necessary for her to seek a third opinion. In view of the frequency of unnecessary procedures, it would seem that the decision to obtain a third opinion may be a very worthwhile one.

Hope for the future

There are multiple abuses occurring in medicine, most of which are the result of economic pressures. The majority of these abuses are the result of unethical practices by a small number of physicians who are, for the most part, uncontrolled by the medical profession and unrecognizable to the consuming public. Besides that, there are many less frequent abuses involving almost the entire medical community. The public must constantly be on the alert to avoid them.

Patients who are careful consumers and who do not accept anything on *blind* trust can make the difference. They can identify and avoid physicians who would take advantage of them. They can be watchdogs of what kinds of treatment are offered. Ultimately, they are the consumers who will force changes in the medical profession which are urgently needed. Eventually, the number of patients who are treated by charlatans will decrease and they will find their way into the hands of honorable physicians who are worthy of their trust.

Realism leads us to understand that neither the medical profession nor any other part of our lives is perfect. But let us never give up seeking that perfection.

INDEX

Page numbers followed by a "t" indicate a table concerning the subject.